Mental Health in Historical Perspective

Series Editors
Catharine Coleborne
School of Humanities and Social Science
University of Newcastle
Callaghan, NSW, Australia

Matthew Smith
Centre for the Social History of Health and Healthcare
University of Strathclyde
Glasgow, UK

Covering all historical periods and geographical contexts, the series explores how mental illness has been understood, experienced, diagnosed, treated and contested. It will publish works that engage actively with contemporary debates related to mental health and, as such, will be of interest not only to historians, but also mental health professionals, patients and policy makers. With its focus on mental health, rather than just psychiatry, the series will endeavour to provide more patient-centred histories. Although this has long been an aim of health historians, it has not been realised, and this series aims to change that.

The scope of the series is kept as broad as possible to attract good quality proposals about all aspects of the history of mental health from all periods. The series emphasises interdisciplinary approaches to the field of study, and encourages short titles, longer works, collections, and titles which stretch the boundaries of academic publishing in new ways.

More information about this series at
http://www.palgrave.com/gp/series/14806

Åsa Jansson

From Melancholia to Depression

Disordered Mood in Nineteenth-Century
Psychiatry

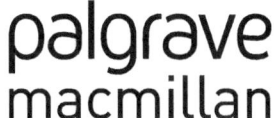

Åsa Jansson
Institute for Medical Humanities
Durham University
Durham, UK

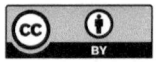

Mental Health in Historical Perspective
ISBN 978-3-030-54801-8   ISBN 978-3-030-54802-5   (eBook)
https://doi.org/10.1007/978-3-030-54802-5

Cover credit: Teodoro Ortiz Tarrascusa/Alamy Stock Photo

This Palgrave Macmillan imprint is published by the registered company Springer Nature Switzerland AG
The registered company address is: Gewerbestrasse 11, 6330 Cham, Switzerland

For Annika. Thank you, for everything.

PREFACE

This book has been a long time in the making. The seeds were sown in 2009 when I started researching an M.A. dissertation on melancholia and depressed mood in Wilhelm Griesinger's work, and quickly realised that there was a much bigger story to be told about what happened to the melancholia concept in nineteenth-century psychiatry. This story became the focus of a Ph.D. thesis on which this book is based.

Melancholia is a topic that has attracted vast attention from writers across disciplines and genres, spanning a range of perspectives. At the same time, much existing work on melancholia is underpinned by a common theme: the belief that melancholy is a timeless human emotion, a phenomenon that has remained largely constant as our societies have changed, a shared experience that connects us to our ancestors of past historical periods. Seen in this way, melancholy is a core feature of humanity, as is its pathological mutation, melancholia. To understand melancholia, then, is to understand something about what it means to be human: to suffer without apparent cause.

As this is the context in which this book is written, and as it will inevitably be read against the backdrop of a large catalogue of works on melancholia and melancholy, it is only right that I confess that my interest in this topic and my original motivation for exploring it are less ambitious and more mundane than those of many of the writers who have sought to make sense of this ubiquitous yet elusive feature of the human condition. My initial interest in mood disorders arose in relation to the politics of the pharmaceutical industry and the medicalisation of psychological distress that provides a lucrative market for drug companies. I once offered this explanation in a scholarship interview, and it didn't go down very well. It was not, it seemed, how or why one is supposed to do history. It was, however, the truth, though that original motivation has since been superseded by a more fundamental desire to understand how knowledge in the psy disciplines is produced, in particular relating to psychiatric classification.

But I was never particularly interested in exploring melancholy as a feeling. In the field of the history of psychiatry, the question that often looms—usually unspoken—over our heads when we talk about our research is that of personal experience. Do you write about melancholia because of your own struggles with pathological low mood? The short answer to that is no. My interest is more broadly in the production of psychiatric knowledge about people, how our emotions, thoughts, and actions become symptoms of psychiatric diagnoses. Depression has become ubiquitous, more so than any other psychiatric condition—the WHO considers it to be a leading cause of disability worldwide and the prescription and consumption of antidepressant medication continue to rise every year. I wanted to understand how we got to this point. But when I delved into the world of historical scholarship on depression and melancholia I soon discovered that a significant piece of the puzzle was missing.

The more I read, the more evident it became that something fundamental occurred in the nineteenth century. Most writers on the topic, whether they subscribe to a narrative of continuity or one of change, recognise that today's Major Depressive Disorder doesn't correspond to past conceptions of melancholia. But nineteenth-century melancholia was not only significantly different from clinical depression as understood today, it was equally different from the various forms of traditional melancholy madness that came before. As German Berrios has noted, a shift occurred that was about more than just a change in language.[1] The reconceptualisation of melancholia in the nineteenth century facilitated the later emergence of clinical depression in the twentieth, but it also paved the

---

[1] German E. Berrios, "Melancholia and Depression during the Nineteenth Century: A Conceptual History," *British Journal of Psychiatry* 153 (1988): 298–304.

way for the creation of other affect-based diagnostic categories, such as bipolar disorder, borderline personality disorder, and anxiety disorders.

The story of how melancholia was reconfigured along biomedical lines is not, then, only the story of a specific diagnosis, or state of mind, it is also the story of how the modern concept 'mood disorder' was created. That story didn't begin on asylum wards, but with the rise of a new discipline: experimental physiology. The epistemological framework that was created in the early nineteenth century to explain the internal operation of emotions and ideas continues to form the basis for how we think about psychological events today, and consequently informs the direction of current research into the mind and brain. If we want to understand how we arrived at this point in history where 'depression' is an illness that can be treated with psychotropic medication and therapeutic strategies aimed at teaching us to 'regulate' our emotions, we must first understand how the idea of disordered mood as a medical condition became possible in the first place. And we must also understand the relationship between statistics and diagnostic practices, another distinctly modern development that is crucial to mapping the creation not just of mood disorders but of most modern psychiatric diagnoses.

This book, then, is an attempt to redress a significant gap in the history of depression and melancholia, and of mood disorders more generally. It arises from a desire to understand how knowledge that is absolutely fundamental to the human experience in the twenty-first century was created and made real. So, I didn't come to this topic because of an interest in melancholy as a feeling or a personal experience with depression. But of course, an interest in psychiatric knowledge is an interest in knowledge about human distress and suffering, and in this way it concerns us all. Most if not all of us will experience psychological distress at some point in our lives (whether or not that distress is pathologised and diagnosed). And what I found once I immersed myself in the archival records of Victorian asylums was that while I don't necessarily relate to twenty-first-century descriptions of clinical depression, some of the ways in which nineteenth-century asylum patients diagnosed with melancholia expressed their distress resonated with me deeply. Many Victorian melancholics appeared to display 'symptoms' that are largely consistent with the key criteria of depression today, but equally common were profound delusions, and in more severe cases hallucinations were not unusual.

This led me to start asking questions about our current separation of affective (mood) and cognitive (schizo) disorders, which began in the nineteenth century and was cemented in the twentieth. That story is yet to be told, and doesn't form part of this book. But it looms in the background and illustrates one of the most important differences between nineteenth-century melancholia and clinical depression, in that delusions and hallucinations are only a secondary and much less talked about feature of the latter.

Finally, it should be emphasised that there are many ways in which one can write the history of nineteenth-century melancholia. This book is an attempt to write it as the history of medical and psychiatric conceptions of what melancholia was—and became—in this period. In other words, this book is not a search for answers about what melancholia feels (or felt) like or why people are apparently afflicted by it. Nor is it an attempt to right historical wrongs in psychiatry by demonstrating the timelessness of melancholia as a medical condition. And it is not a critique of the ubiquity of the clinical depression concept. These are all important issues, which to various extents form the context for the present story, but they have been, and are still being, comprehensively discussed elsewhere. This book is the story of how the first modern mood disorder was created.

Why is this important? There are undoubtedly many reasons, but the most fundamental is this: 'knowledge about human beings changes what people are'.[2] An historical perspective on such knowledge is crucial. It allows us to understand where it comes from, how it emerged, how it operates, and most importantly how it becomes central to our lives. It shows us that such knowledge is not permanent or universal. Mood disorders constitute a particular, historically specific way of making sense of and experiencing emotional distress. What shedding light on this historical specificity does is show us that the existence of this framework is not inevitable. It's very much real today—people are diagnosed with mood disorders and experience themselves as suffering from these conditions—but it hasn't always been. This way of understanding emotional distress is neither right nor wrong; it can be both helpful and harmful. What is important is that we are equipped with the tools to think critically about its place in our lives and the work that it does, and to equally allow for

---

[2] Roger Smith, *Being Human: Historical Knowledge and the Creation of Human Nature* (Manchester: Manchester University Press, 2007), 8.

different frameworks and ways of experience. This, in my view, is one of the most important tasks of history: to remind us of the impermanence of human nature, and that we have the power to fundamentally change the way we understand our inner selves and the world around us.

Durham, UK   Åsa Jansson

Acknowledgements

I'm indebted to many people and institutions for their help and support in the research and writing of this book. Thanks first of all to Molly Beck at Palgrave Macmillan for her enthusiastic interest in and support for the book, as well as to Maeve Sinnott for continuous support and guidance during the writing process. Thanks also to the editors of the *Mental Health in Historical Perspective* series, Catharine Coleborne and Matthew Smith, and to the anonymous peer reviewers for their helpful comments on the proposal and manuscript.

This book would not have been possible without a generous scholarship from the Wellcome Trust (grant number 092988/Z/10/Z), which allowed me to research and write the thesis on which the book is based. I'm also grateful to my colleagues and friends at the University of London whose feedback at various stages of this project in its early years was instrumental in shaping the story that eventually became the present book, in particular my Ph.D. supervisors Thomas Dixon and Rhodri Hayward, as well as Sarah Chaney, Chris Millard, Jennifer Wallis, Tom Quick, Stephen Jacyna, and Sonu Shamdasani. I'm also especially grateful to Felicity Callard for continuous support and advice over the years.

Thanks also to my colleagues at the Institute for Medical Humanities and Hearing the Voice at Durham University, in particular Angela Woods, Sarah Atkinson, Victoria Patton, Ben Alderson-Day, Chris Cook, Charles Fernyhough, Kaja Mitrenga, and Mary Robson. Working in a collaborative and interdisciplinary context over the last few years has had a profound impact on my approach to history, and has led me to ask sometimes difficult and uncomfortable questions about the role of historical research and historical perspective in the medical humanities, and more fundamentally in our common endeavour to understand and redress human suffering.

I'm also grateful to the following people for feedback, advice, and/or fruitful conversations that have provided insight and guidance over the years since I first began researching this topic: Ingrid Lindstedt, Roger Smith, Rob Iliffe, Roger Cooter, Rebecca O'Neal, Victoria O'Callaghan, Yewande Okuleye, and Eric Engstrom, as well as everyone who has offered questions and comments on seminar and conference talks based on different aspects of this research.

Finally, my deepest gratitude is due to the people whose unconditional love and support have kept me (relatively) sane through the various stages of this journey: Annika, Annelie, Britta, Melek, Becky, Shannon, Anna, Danny, Sophie, Hanna, and Olly. Thank you.

CONTENTS

CONTENTS

CHAPTER 1

Introduction: Disordered Mood as Historical Problem

If mania and melancholia took on the face that we still recognise today, it is not because we have learnt to 'open our eyes' to their real nature during the course of the centuries; and it is not because we have purified our perceptive processes until they became transparent. It is because in the experience of madness, these concepts were integrated around specific qualitative themes that have lent them their own unity and given them a significant coherence, finally rendering them perceptible.[1]

Michel Foucault, *History of Madness* (1961)

In the summer of 1874, Moses B., a young doctor, was brought into Edinburgh Royal Asylum at Morningside. According to his family, he had become so intent on taking his own life that they saw no other option but to have him certified as insane and admitted to the hospital. One of the doctors who examined him in his home had written in the medical certificate that Moses suffered from severe 'delusions', which had him convinced that 'his soul is lost, that he ought to die' and that 'he is committing great sins'. When Moses arrived at Morningside, the attending physician noted in the patient journal that the young man's 'depression' was 'considerable', and made a note of his 'suicidal tendencies', which, based on family testimony, consisted in 'taking belladonna, refusing food, &c'. Moses B. was subsequently diagnosed with melancholia, with emphasis given to his pronounced 'suicidal tendencies', which required that he be placed under close observation.

© The Author(s) 2021
Å Jansson, *From Melancholia to Depression,*
Mental Health in Historical Perspective,
https://doi.org/10.1007/978-3-030-54802-5_1

1

For the experienced medical staff at Morningside, diagnosing Moses was a straightforward matter. Melancholia was, at the time, a common affliction among patients who arrived in the asylum. Its symptoms were considered to be clearly recognisable and, according to the institution's chief physician, Thomas Clouston, the disease ran 'a somewhat definite course, like a fever'.[2] But what would a twenty-first-century psychiatrist or general practitioner make of a patient like Moses Black? Would they conclude that he suffered from Major Depressive Disorder, prescribe him a course of antidepressants, and put him on the waiting list for Cognitive Behavioural Therapy? Or would his thoughts and actions—believing himself to have sinned against God and attempting to poison himself—appear unfamiliar to today's clinicians? These questions speak to a more profound, ontological concern: is clinical depression a timeless condition? In other words, have people always been depressed?

I will return to this question momentarily. Whether or not depression has always been a feature of the human condition, if current statistics are to be believed we are, as a society, becoming more depressed with each passing year. According to the World Health Organisation, clinical depression is now the world's leading cause of disability. When a new generation of antidepressant drugs, selective serotonin reuptake inhibitors (SSRIs), flooded the market in the late twentieth century, one scholar suggested that we had entered an 'antidepressant era'.[3] In the 1990s, SSRIs became what benzodiazepines were to the sixties—the universal cure for unwanted negative emotions. A common question in response to these developments, which has been posed by scholars across the natural and human sciences, is whether rates of depression have increased, or whether we have become less tolerant of emotional distress, or simply more likely to denote it as a medical problem with a chemical solution. It has been suggested that the apparent rise in depression is primarily due to a growing tendency to over-diagnose 'normal sadness'.[4] Others argue that there has been a real increase in the symptoms of genuine Major Depressive Disorder since the early twentieth century, leading one observer to conclude that depression is, like obesity and type-II diabetes, a 'disease of modernity' caused by humanity's collective derailment from our true evolutionary path, suggesting that 'humans have dragged a body with a long hominid history into an overfed, malnourished, sedentary, sunlight-deficient, sleep-deprived, competitive, inequitable, and socially-isolating environment with dire consequences'.[5]

However, a different school of thought exists that has found support both in clinical circles and among some humanities scholars: that, historically, two types of depression have coexisted.[6] One is a mild to moderate form of mood disorder, what is usually meant by the term 'clinical depression' today: low mood and sadness, often accompanied by sleeplessness, appetite disruption, and anxiety. The other is an endogenous form that is more than a mental disorder, it is an illness where the entire system is, in effect, 'pressed down', resulting in retarded speech and slow bodily movement. This illness often manifests with delusions (psychosis) and can in its most severe forms leave sufferers in a catatonic stupor. This condition is usually referred to as psychotic or melancholic depression. Existing research on this type of depression holds the promise of something that has eluded psychiatry since its infancy: a mood disorder with a traceable and measurable biological basis. Endocrine psychiatry indicates that individuals who fit the external symptomatology for melancholic depression show similar results when subjected to a Dexamethasone Suppression Test (DST) measuring the level of cortisol in the blood. Such research is, however, marginalised in the current neuro-focused climate where neurotransmitters are conceptualised as the cause, effect, and cure for depression, and where the major diagnostic manuals retain a descriptive focus. Another key feature of melancholic depression is its perceived resistance to standard antidepressant treatments such as SSRIs and behavioural therapies; instead, it is argued that patients tend to respond to a combination of electroconvulsive therapy and atypical (tricyclic) antidepressants. In recent years, a number of scholars and clinicians have sought to institute this type of depression into diagnostic literature as an illness in its own right: melancholia.[7]

This drive to formally institute melancholia into psychiatric diagnostic literature is presented as an attempted 'resurrection' of a condition that has existed throughout human history and been documented by physicians as far back as Hippocrates. This melancholia, its proponents argue, 'lends itself to definition as an independent entity in the classification' and 'is consistent with centuries of observation'.[8] It is constituted as universal and timeless, the 'real' depression, whereas our time's standard clinical depression is seen to have more in common with the nervous disorders of the early modern period or neurasthenia in the nineteenth century. Authors beyond the psy disciplines who have adopted this view constitute a broad church, including historians, philosophers, and social scientists, and their work is prominent within existing scholarship on the history of melancholia.[9]

Max Fink and Michael Taylor, two psychiatrists who are at the forefront of the campaign to resurrect melancholia, argue that this disease is 'consistently' described in 'psychopathological literature' as 'a severe illness of acute onset with unremitting moods of apprehension and gloom, psychomotor disturbance, and vegetative signs. Psychosis, intermittent mania, and suicide intent are prominent features'.[10] What is most noteworthy about this is not the definition itself, but that the 'psychopathological literature' referred to is from the mid-nineteenth century. Indeed, while those attempting to 'resurrect' melancholia assert that this illness has existed since the beginning of time, the disease they are seeking to revive appears to be an updated version of a diagnostic category specific to nineteenth-century psychological medicine.

What, then, is this nineteenth-century melancholia that some writers are attempting to bring back to life? Is it a timeless illness finally discovered and described by nineteenth-century doctors? It would certainly be possible to write the history of melancholic depression as the history of a medical condition that has existed since the dawn of humanity, and which was finally given an accurate scientific description in the nineteenth century. But this narrative ignores a number of important factors. First of all, the very idea of a 'mood disorder' was not possible before a modern, scientific model of emotion was created. Secondly, melancholic depression was not suddenly discovered with the help of modern medical science. Rather, the meaning of melancholia as a medical condition changed—in other words, melancholia was reconceptualised as a modern mood disorder in the nineteenth century. This process required significant intellectual work, and was made possible by the appropriation of experimental physiology to talk about unseen and unmeasurable mental phenomena. The model of emotion that emerged in the early-to-mid-nineteenth century was not *discovered*, it was *made*—originally as an analogy of sensory-motor action, which eventually became a scientific concept in its own right. There was nothing inevitable about this development; as one scholar has suggested, 'implications had to be *constructed* rather than merely extrapolated'.[11] Finally, as will be demonstrated in the chapters that follow, the melancholia that was described by nineteenth-century physicians and diagnosed in asylum patients had a distinct symptomatology, which does not seamlessly correspond to either the milder or the 'melancholic' depressions that are diagnosed today.

There exists, then, a different history of melancholia and depression, one that is yet to be told. It is this history that is the focus of this book. It maps the first decades of melancholia as a biomedical disease, but rather than showing how this timeless illness was finally discovered and correctly described by modern psychiatry, this book tells the story of how the idea of a 'mood disorder' was created in the nineteenth century and subsequently made into a possible and plausible medical concept. This was a development that to some extent occurred simultaneously in several European countries; however, important national differences existed. For instance, French physicians were more concerned with melancholia as one stage of 'circular insanity' (the other being mania) than their German or British counterparts; indeed, British physicians held that cases of circular insanity were rare among their patients. Such geographical differences speak to the malleability of mental disorders not just across time, but also across cultural or linguistic contexts. This book is primarily concerned with melancholia in the British context, for three reasons. First of all, melancholia was consistently diagnosed in British asylums throughout the second half of the nineteenth century, and the wealth of asylum records and statistical reports, as well as prolific diagnostic literature on melancholia, offer an optimal space for interrogating this medical category. In many asylums across the country, melancholia was the second most common diagnosis after mania. From the mid-nineteenth century onward, the rate increased gradually, and at the same time, the diagnosis was gradually standardised. This coherence across asylums as far apart as Edinburgh and Sussex was in part the result of a standardised regime imposed by the Lunacy Commission from the 1840s onward, as well as growing professional interaction between asylum physicians through meetings and publications. Secondly, Germany is often presented in historical narratives as the cradle of modern psychiatric knowledge and the most important influence on contemporary diagnostics. This is in part due to the significance of Emil Kraepelin's work and the prominent place awarded to his nosology in both historical and contemporary texts on psychiatric diagnostics. However, while Kraepelin's division of mental disorders into dementia praecox and manic-depressive insanity at the turn of the twentieth century had a fundamental impact on the subsequent classification of insanity, his diagnostic system was the product and articulation of decades of accumulated knowledge, much of which originated within British psychological medicine. In particular, one of the most

crucial developments of modern psychiatry and the focus of this book—
the creation of 'mood disorder' as a medical category—can in large
part be attributed to the intellectual context of British asylum medicine.
Finally, while a truly inter- or transcultural history of melancholia in this
period would no doubt be a fascinating one, such an approach would limit
the possibility for an in-depth study of its transformation. At the same
time, however, the making of melancholia as a modern mood disorder
in Victorian medicine did not occur in a national vacuum. The uptake of
German and, to an extent, French medical knowledge into British psychological medicine was instrumental, and consequently forms part of the
present story.

This book begins with early nineteenth-century experimental physiology and ends in the Victorian asylum at the turn of the twentieth
century. Victorian physicians conceptualised melancholia as a form of
affective insanity in which the intellect was left wholly or partially intact.
During European psychiatry's foundational century biological disease
models came to dominate, underpinned by increasingly refined medico-
scientific technology, specifically microscopy. Physicians were able to 'see'
into the brains of deceased patients in ways never before possible, and
eagerly searched for cerebral lesions to support biomedical theories of
mental disease. Contrary to one historian's suggestion that 'neuropsy-
chiatry never really flourished in Britain',[12] Victorian medical psychologists embraced neurological explanatory frameworks for mental disease.
However, despite the spread and growing sophistication of psychiatric
autopsies in Europe, some forms of madness consistently failed to turn
up visible changes to brain tissue.[13] This was particularly the case with
milder forms of insanity where the emotions were seen as the chief site
of pathology. In a biomedical context, such illness came to be explained
primarily through functional physiological (rather than structural anatomical) language.

In 1883, Scottish asylum physician Thomas Clouston defined melancholia as 'mental pain, emotional depression, and sense of ill-being,
usually more intense than in melancholy, with loss of self-control, or
insane delusions, or uncontrollable impulses towards suicide, with no
proper capacity left to follow ordinary avocations, with some of the
ordinary interests of life destroyed, and generally with marked bodily
symptoms'.[14] At this time, melancholia was not only one of the most
common forms of mental disease diagnosed in British asylums, it was also
one of the most standardised and homogenous diagnoses, both in terms

of a coherent symptom picture and an internal biological explanatory model. Yet only a few decades earlier, the nosological status of melancholia in British (and European) medicine was unclear and unstable, with some of the most prominent medical writers trying to do away with this category altogether. Its symptomatology was similarly far more diverse and inconsistent in the first half of the nineteenth century, often overlapping with other conditions such as monomania and moral insanity. Thus, while the term melancholia had been used to denote a form of illness or madness in medical literature since antiquity, the biomedical model of melancholia that emerged in the mid-nineteenth century was historically new and conceptually different from any earlier meanings of the term.

Two developments in particular were foundational to this new model of melancholia. The first was the uptake of physiological language and concepts into psychological medicine. In the early decades of the nineteenth century, physicians began to appropriate language from experimental physiology to speak about the perceived internal operations of ideas and emotions. Such models became central to the development of modern psychiatric concepts, particularly that of disordered mood. The emergence of what became known as physiological psychology and its significance for mid-to-late nineteenth-century conceptions of mind have been considered in detail elsewhere.[15] The role of physiological models of mental pathology in the creation of modern mood disorders is, however, largely absent from the history of psychiatry. The reconfiguration of melancholia as a biomedical disease and a form of affective insanity was dependent upon the creation of 'disordered emotion' as a medical category. It follows that in order to adequately map the evolution of nineteenth-century melancholia one must trace how the idea of disordered and pathological emotionality was constituted and appropriated by medical psychologists to speak about mental disease.

The second key development was the institutionalisation of medical statistics together with a standardisation of recording practices in asylums across Britain. Following the creation of the Lunacy Commission in 1845, diagnostic practices were increasingly carried out within an administrative framework heavily reliant upon asylum statistics. While historians of psychiatry have made considerable use of asylum statistics in constructing various narratives, both local and on a wider geographical scale, the relationship between such numerical data and the creation of an increasing number of diagnostic categories in nineteenth-century psychological medicine has been curiously neglected. As I demonstrate in Chapters 5 and 6 of this book, statistical and recording practices were crucial in shaping melancholia as a modern diagnostic category. In sum, nineteenth-century melancholia was constituted through the interplay between the language of physiological psychology, statistical practices, and clinical diagnostics, which together facilitated the creation of a modern biomedical disease concept.

Central to the developments described above was the use of metaphorical language to explain mental operations.[16] As a form of affective insanity, melancholia was a disease perceived to rarely leave internal marks on patients' brain tissue. Through the application of metaphors borrowed from experimental physiology, such as 'irritation', 'reflex', and 'tone', disordered emotion could be explained as a defective physiological process. Moreover, the biomedical language of physiology contributed to a conceptual and linguistic shift in the description of external 'symptoms' of melancholia. Symptoms such as 'depression' and 'mental pain' (or 'psychalgia') rose to prominence in the second half of the nineteenth century. These terms have a history that pre-dates modern scientific medicine. Within the framework of a physiologically constituted model of mental pathology, older terms were imbued with new meanings. The language used by medical writers to explain mental phenomena is central to the present story, and the semantic ambivalence of medico-psychological terminology will gradually unfold in the subsequent chapters.

A Note on Language

While much of the medical and scientific terminology of the nineteenth century sounds familiar to the twenty-first reader, familiarity does not equate to sameness. This book attempts to strike a balance between contextual and historical sensitivity on the one hand, and rendering Victorian concepts intelligible in twenty-first-century language on the other. With that in mind, two words in particular that feature throughout this book warrant clarification.

1. *Biomedical*. Geneticists Craig Venter and Daniel Cohen have referred to the twenty-first century as 'the century of biology'.[17] This pronouncement is perhaps a little premature, but what is more certain is that, over the last century and a half, biology has become central to how we understand ourselves and the world around us. In its modern meaning, that is, the way it gradually came to be used from the nineteenth century onward, biology is, broadly speaking, 'the science of life'.[18] The scientists

and doctors whose work is discussed in this book were concerned with the study of living organisms, a category that included human beings. It follows that many of the medical events and phenomena described in this book are referred to as biological. The organism–environment dualism emerged in this period and emotion was believed to be produced in the brain through the interaction—and disequilibrium—between the two. To describe melancholia in the mid-to-late nineteenth century as biological would, however, suggest only part of the picture. The condition was facilitated by the fusion of the new experimental sciences with medical knowledge, and is consequently referred to here as *biomedical*.

Biomedicine and its adjective did not come into use in the English language until the 1920s,[19] in other words, some two decades after the conclusion of the present story. Why, then, use it to describe nineteenth-century melancholia in a narrative that explicitly emphasises the importance of historical context and specificity? Following Clarke et al., I use 'biomedical' to denote 'the increasingly biological scientific aspects of the practices of clinical medicine'.[20] While the term biomedical belongs to the twentieth and twenty-first centuries, the process it refers to began in the nineteenth. In the mid-to-late nineteenth century, melancholia was reconstituted along biological (primarily physiological) lines, and it was conceptualised as a disorder of emotion, bringing the latter within the purview of medical science in new ways. As will be seen in the story that unfolds, Victorian physicians became increasingly concerned with non-delusional affective insanity as well as with emotional disturbances not considered strictly pathological. This constituted a profound shift (or shifts) in perceptions of human life, of medicine, and of the health/illness dichotomy. When I began to research this book, I needed an adjective for this new melancholia that emerged, one that would encompass these developments and denote the distinctly modern quality of this disease concept. Moreover, while this book is concerned with historical specificity and change, it is just as much about continuity. Specifically, the continuity of a macro-ontology of emotion as a biological operation (physiological and automated) subject to medical interrogation. This definition of emotion was created through the appropriation of data from experimental physiology, an area of research that utilised new technologies and techniques to study the animal body. Situated within this framework, melancholia was construed in modern, scientific terms radically different from pre-nineteenth-century descriptions of melancholy madness. It became, in short, a new disease. Referring to this melancholia as 'biomedical' is intended to highlight this significant conceptual shift, in language familiar to the twenty-first-century reader.

2. *Depression.* Scholars writing histories of melancholia or melancholy have often done so under the assumption that underlying cultural and temporal differences in language and understanding is a more or less timeless condition, a mood disorder that corresponds largely to what is today known as clinical depression. At the same time, as suggested above, critics of the twenty-first-century model of depression that appears to grow increasingly inclusive and opaque, have turned to past descriptions of melancholia in an attempt to show that there exists a core condition— a severe form of depression usually accompanied by psychosis—that has remained relatively stable across time, but which is becoming eclipsed by the current fashion of extending the term depression to an increasingly wide range of emotional states. These different but overlapping perceptions of melancholia and depression make it difficult to write a history of the former without also taking the latter into consideration. However, while it is important to acknowledge that a close link exists between nineteenth-century melancholia and the depressions of the twentieth and twenty-first centuries, the nature of this relationship should not be taken for granted. There is no inevitable and uncontested historical trajectory that leads from one to the other—such a linear development has been read and written into the histories of melancholia and depression by the people writing such histories.

'Depression' has been used unproblematically to speak about mental suffering in the eighteenth and nineteenth centuries.[21] This is not simply a question of historians projecting modern terminology onto a past where it did not exist. The use of the term depression to denote a low mental state, such as profound sadness, has featured in the English language at least since the mid-seventeenth century. In this way, it was a metaphorical description of a mind or soul 'pressed down'; close in meaning to its literal, geometrical sense.[22] In Victorian psychological medicine, 'depression' was reconstituted within the repertoire of words with strong physiological connotations, such as 'irritation', 'cerebral reflex', and 'tone'. In this context, it was equally used to denote low mood, but in a more literal (physical) sense than today, since the physiological framework allowed for a perception of mental functioning as lowered or slowed down. This phenomenon was often linked to decreased blood flow to the brain, and consequently impaired cerebral nutrition. Due to the multifaceted history of the term, it is difficult to pin down the medical roots of depression as a psychiatric symptom; however, its nineteenth-century meaning may have been at least partially appropriated from cardiovascular medicine.[23] Depression used in this way became a key symptom of melancholia alongside 'mental pain' and 'suicidal tendencies'. It was also used as an umbrella category for various states of affective insanity characterised by low mood, often referred to as the 'states of mental depression', contrasted with the 'states of mental weakness' and the 'states of mental exaltation'. However, it is important to note that Victorian physicians did not speak of depression as a mental disease or disorder. Prior to the twentieth century, depression was a symptom or a unifying descriptive term, but it was not understood as a specific medical condition. Nineteenth-century usage of the word was more semantically different from ours than is generally acknowledged today. The tendency to equate nineteenth-century melancholia with today's depression can at least in part be attributed to a lack of contextual and semantic sensitivity displayed by scholars when using the term depression in pre-twentieth-century narratives.[24]

MELANCHOLY AND MELANCHOLIA BEFORE THE NINETEENTH CENTURY

While depression is, then, a strictly modern illness category, melancholia has a long history as a medical condition (or, rather, conditions), going back as far as the origins of the word, which derives from the Greek μέλας (*melas*) and χολή (*kholé*), meaning 'black bile'.[25] The various forms of ancient, medieval, and early modern melancholias should not be grouped into one uniform, pre-modern category; nevertheless, Angus Gowland notes that '[i]n terms of medical theory, the history of melancholy from antiquity to early modernity is predominantly one of continuity rather than change'.[26] Taken together, these classical forms of melancholy or melancholia stand in stark contrast to the melancholia of the mid-to-late nineteenth century. Earlier versions, taken as a group, had strong links to the gastric region (as a result of the humoural hypothesis on which the disease concept was based), and were generally characterised by vivid delusions and a profound and debilitating sadness.[27] While contemporary historians have referred to classical forms of melancholia as a 'mental disorder',[28] it was not universally understood as a form of madness; medical and theological explanations often conflicted over its nature. Melancholy could be a temperament, a persona, a religious sentiment, or a sorrowful state of mind (or soul). Melancholia as a disease was, like other forms of illness, a humoural imbalance, believed to result from an excess of black bile. When the bile overflowed and rose to the head, clouding the mind and soul, this would produce sadness, fear, and delusions. In this regard it was often, but not always, perceived as 'a species of madness (delirium) involving the impairment of a principal internal mental faculty, and usually accompanied by groundless fear and sorrow'.[29]

Despite numerous palpable similarities across centuries, the many pre-modern melancholias equally took on various distinct features specific to the cultural and temporal context of each form. Among early medieval monks, for instance, a prominent feature of melancholy and melancholia was acedia, 'a condition that particularly affected hermit monks in the desert'.[30] Acedia was a negative, indifferent state of mind, in which one had little interest in or concern for one's surroundings. Described in fourth-century literature as a hatred of the present moment and a profound desire to be somewhere else, it was caused by the demon of acedia, also known as the 'middle of the day demon' from its tendency to appear during the hottest hours of the day among the monks who lived in desert colonies outside Alexandria.[31] During the Baroque period, conversely, melancholy chiefly affected men of great artistry and intel-lectual abilities, and could result in terrifying delusions, such as the 'glass man' (believing oneself to be made of glass and thus fearful of being shat-tered into thousands of pieces). Other such early modern experiences of melancholy included the self-perception of being part man and part wolf, wild and uncontrollable (the 'wolf man'—a delusion given meaning and reality through popular stories about werewolves), as well as the sensation of being made entirely out of butter (thus prone to melt in the sun), or from straw (thus unable to stand up).[32] In eighteenth-century England, melancholy became 'the English malady', an affliction primarily affecting persons of the upper classes whose 'nerves' were weak, and which was often linked to the cold, damp climate of the British Isles, as well as to the sedentary lifestyle of the landed gentry.[33] This nervous affliction, overlap-ping with the 'vapours' and 'spleen', should be distinguished from the late nineteenth-century affliction 'nervous exhaustion' (or 'neurasthenia'), a condition brought on by a combination of the ills of modern urban life and too much 'brain work'.[34]

THE CHANGING FACE OF MELANCHOLIA

As these historical vignettes indicate, melancholia is not, and never has been, one thing. The meaning of the word has changed over time, sometimes significantly, and other words have equally been used to describe emotional states that we might today associate with melancholia. For over two thousand years, doctors, philosophers, scientists, theologians, historians, artists, and writers have tried to make sense of low mood, in particular the shifting and often opaque boundary between health and illness. Anyone attempting to write a history of melancholia, whether as a form of madness, an emotion, a temperament, an artistic trope, or as depression previously called by a different name will, intentionally or not, add their story to a vast catalogue of scholarship spanning all of these perspectives, sometimes brought together in a single narrative.[35] As the existing body of work on the history of melancholia attests, scholars continue to be drawn to the topic, attempting to understand where contemporary experiences of low mood fit in the wider context of human history. Our ability to experience profound and at times debilitating emotional depression appears to be a feature that unites the human species across temporal and cultural boundaries. At the same time, the range of experiences associated with melancholy, melancholia, and depression suggest that these psychological states come in an endless number of different shades and nuances.

To capture in a single narrative the multitude of imagery that is conjured up by the melancholia term is no easy feat, and it is harder yet to create order among this chaos of emotionality. One writer who has managed this with considerable skill and success is intellectual historian Karin Johannisson, whose history of melancholy is an apt illustration of its multifaceted nature. She maps some of the different ways in which low mood has been conceptualised and experienced in different societies in the West, showing how emotional expressions associated with melancholy have changed over time. In doing so she asks whether 'each epoch generates its own emotional repertoire'.[36] While Johannisson suggests that hers is a history of the emotions rather than of medicine, she nonetheless draws heavily on medical sources in order to contextualise the 'experience' of melancholy, testifying to the difficulty in making any definitive distinction between medical condition and emotion. Her history of melancholy is, then, also a history of melancholia and of depression, which attempts to organise and differentiate types of melancholic qualities associated with different historical periods. Johannisson does this by separating low mood into three, temporally anchored, shades of melancholy: black (early modern), grey (modern), and white (late modern). All three are presented in fragments, medical and popular notions intermingled and boundaries obscured. This mosaic presentation of what is at one moment a feeling and at the next a medical condition is poignant and aptly illustrative of how meanings attached to the terms melancholy, melancholia, and depression have not only changed over time, but how different and even conflicting notions of these concepts have often coexisted.

Broadly speaking, existing histories of melancholia can be divided into two camps: one emphasising continuity, the other historical specificity and change.[37] Johannisson's study exemplifies the latter, while Stanley Jackson's comprehensive work on melancholia and depression through the ages takes a continuity perspective. *Melancholia and Depression: From Hippocratic Times to Modern Times*, first published in 1986, remains the most ambitious attempt to date to piece together a coherent history of low mood spanning more than two millennia. Jackson frames his narrative as the history of depressive illness, suggesting that this condition, traditionally known as melancholia, has shown 'both a remarkable consistency and a remarkable coherence in the basic cluster of symptoms' across time.[38] More recently, Clark Lawlor has attempted a similarly expansive history that traces melancholia from ancient Greece to the twenty-first century. Lawlor laments the end of a centuries-old continuity with the 'paradigm-changing arrival' of the third edition of the American Psychiatric Association's *Diagnostic and Statistical Manual of Mental Disorders (DSM-III)* in 1980, which produced a new depression based solely on descriptive psychopathology and which expanded into the realm of normal sadness.[39] Edward Shorter is similarly critical of the *DSM* approach to mood disorders. He argues for the existence of two distinct forms of depression, one that is endogenous (melancholia), and a socially and culturally produced category, what is today the main form of depressive illness diagnosed in primary care.[40]

Contrasting these narratives with a focus weighted towards historical change, Judith Misbach and Henderikus Stam have traced a conceptual shift in the nineteenth century whereby melancholia was 'gradually reconceptualized as depression' through a process of 'medicalization'.[41] While their study is limited and places particular focus on the relationship between melancholia and neurasthenia, it forms an important contribution to the history of depressed mood. Their narrative follows on from German Berrios, who emphasises the role of French alienist Esquirol's idiosyncratic term *lymemanie* ('sadness mania') in the reconfiguration from intellectual to emotional insanity, arguing that, while the term was only ever used by French and Spanish physicians, it nonetheless helped bring about a change in meaning of the term melancholia, before the latter became gradually replaced by depression. For Berrios, there is little conceptual difference between late nineteenth-century melancholia and early twentieth-century depression. It is primarily a terminological change in large part driven by a preference for the latter term as it 'evoked a "physiological" explanation'.[42] As these narratives imply, there was no straightforward transition from melancholia to depression—the former was not simply replaced by the latter. However, within existing histories tracing the reconfiguration of the melancholia concept in the nineteenth century, two events that were fundamental for this development have been almost completely overlooked. As I demonstrate in the chapters that follow, the shift in psychiatric knowledge relating to depressed mood was underpinned and driven by on the one hand the appropriation of language and concepts from experimental physiology to talk about emotion as a physiological event, and on the other by the role of asylum statistics in the development of diagnostic categories and criteria.

Existing histories of melancholia and depression such as those briefly outlined above testify to the historical instability of these medical concepts, which is foregrounded in Matthew Bell's cultural history of melancholia prior to the nineteenth century. Bell brings attention to the question of whether psychiatric disorders are natural kinds, which in turn speaks to problem of retrospective diagnosis. These issues are at the heart of debates about the relationship between pre-twentieth-century melancholia and today's depressive disorders.[43] Since the nineteenth century, psychiatry's proponents and practitioners have not been averse to reading pre-modern accounts of various afflictions through the spectacles of modern medicine. For instance, Victorian physicians diagnosed Shakespeare's Hamlet with melancholia,[44] twentieth-century psychiatrists have given World War I soldiers PTSD,[45] and medieval saints have been described as schizophrenic.[46] Historians, too, have jumped on this bandwagon, to a lesser degree.[47] The basic premise of this perspective is that categories of classification have changed, but the illnesses to which they refer have remained largely the same across time.

The interlinked questions of retrospective diagnosis and natural kinds in psychiatry illustrate the perpetual tensions that characterise the historical study of illness, particularly of the psychiatric kind, between the universalist and the context-specific, and between the real and the constructed. Following Dominic Murphy, Bell rejects the 'false dichotomy' between 'mental disorders as natural kinds and mental disorders as socially constructed', arguing that psychiatric conditions 'with an organic component can very well have social causes too'.[48] One might argue that there is also a more profound epistemological concern at the core of this debate, as the conceptual distinction between 'organic' and 'social' is historically specific to the modern period. Bracketing this question, however, I agree with Bell that there is no meaningful knowledge to be gained by asking whether or not melancholia is a real or constructed condition. All psychiatric conditions are constructed in the sense that the labels and the clusters of symptoms they refer to are not inevitable or discovered, they are the product of significant intellectual work (which in this book is taken to include a host of clinical and administrative practices and concerns, as well as the theoretical development of diagnostic categories). At the same time, psychiatric conditions are also very much real, insofar as people are diagnosed with them and experience themselves as suffering from such illnesses (this, I would argue, is what makes a psychiatric condition real, irrespective of any perceived organic cause). It follows that in the period with which this book is concerned, melancholia was very much a real condition. But while melancholia has existed as a medical term for over two millennia, the biomedical illness which that term came to denote in the nineteenth century was historically new. The aim of this book is to show how this condition was produced, that is, how melancholia was made into a modern biomedical mood disorder in the nineteenth century—how it was created, shaped, modified, and reified. In other words, it maps the events whereby this particular conception of melancholia was made real.[49]

MELANCHOLIA AND THE HISTORY OF PSYCHIATRY

Why study diagnostic practices? What is the value of such history? Michel Foucault remarked that diagnostic categories are not important in psychiatric medicine. The question is 'not whether it is this or that form of madness, but whether it is or it is not madness'. Everything else is little more than window dressing, an attempt by psychological medicine to resemble more closely its organic counterpart, indeed to *be* organic medicine, rather than to be like it.[50] Psychiatric diagnoses are undoubtedly unstable, fluid, and contingent. But this is precisely why it is so important to subject them to scrutiny and critique. Diagnosis was paramount in nineteenth-century psychological medicine. Medical literature in the second half of the century devoted an extraordinary amount of attention to the difficult act of classifying various forms of mental disease. Each type of illness had to be distinguished from other forms as well as from non-pathological mental states. To be insane was not simply to be delusional.

Existing studies of madness and the asylum in the nineteenth century have contributed much to our understanding of institutionalisation and bureaucracy, and of the everyday practices of psychological medicine. Such histories have made intelligible the Victorian asylum, that odd, foreign place where a struggling profession attempted to treat a range of maladies that were poorly understood and for which there appeared to be few, if any, targeted cures. Much has been made of the struggle of a nascent psychiatric profession to assert itself, to prove its usefulness to society in general and the medical sciences in particular.[51] There exists today a vast and rich catalogue of scholarship addressing the social and political history of psychiatry. Whether concerned with the ways in which power structures were reproduced and reinforced through psychiatric knowledge and institutions,[52] or whether attempting to restore the patient as the protagonist of psychiatric history,[53] social histories of madness and of the asylum have challenged traditional, clinically oriented and largely positivist narratives.[54]

The detailed and comprehensive records that British asylum staff were required to keep on their patients and institutions have provided historians with a wealth of rich source material on individual asylums as well as on the national lunacy bureaucracy. In-depth asylum studies have highlighted local practices and concerns in the context of a wider system in which asylums were increasingly subject to central directives and guidelines. Studies such as Joseph Melling and Bill Forsythe's compelling narrative of the Devon county asylums describe and interrogate the development of clinical knowledge and practices as well as the physical space of the asylum and life within its walls.[55] Until recently, however, the ways in which these spaces and practices were productive of specific kinds of knowledge about mental disease have received limited attention,[56] and the role played by asylum statistics in the creation and consolidation of psychiatric categories remains underresearched.[57] Nevertheless, while diagnostics and classification have rarely been the central focus of existing asylum studies,[58] they have featured as part of broader narratives. For instance, Melling and Forsythe note the high prevalence of melancholia in the Devon county asylums, as well as concerns among staff over the treatment of suicidal patients, who were placed on a 'special ward where attendants could be vigilant at night'.[59]

The picture in the South-West of England was mirrored elsewhere in the country. The number of people admitted to asylums in Britain and diagnosed with melancholia rose sharply in the second half of the nineteenth century, and the management of suicidal patients posed a growing challenge for asylum staff and lunacy commissioners alike. Several physicians noted that the number of melancholic patients increased at a higher rate than admissions overall, prompting discussions over whether more people were suffering from low mood than in the past, or whether such individuals were more likely than previously to be admitted into the asylum. Melancholic patients were rarely seen as posing a danger to others, but they were often believed to be a danger to themselves. The late nineteenth century saw a growing tendency to label melancholics as suicidal on medical certificates, but as discussed in Chapters 5 and 6, the meaning of 'suicidal' was ambiguous. Nevertheless, asylum physicians were increasingly concerned with the correct description and diagnosis of melancholia, and tried to the best of their abilities to identify, label, and categorise the multitude of expressions and behaviours met within their patients and which were seen as indicative of melancholic illness.

The history of melancholia in this period is, then, not just the history of psychiatric knowledge, but also of asylum practices, and of the range of human activity that was read by physicians as signs of melancholia. From the often hastily scribbled notes in asylum casebooks, the twenty-first-century reader catches a glimpse of the human suffering that was translated into diagnostic terms such as 'depressed mood', 'suicidal tendencies', and 'religious delusions'. Snippet quotations tell of people haunted by oppressive feelings of guilt and shame, people who feared that their sins were so grave that they had forfeited the right to live, people who believed themselves persecuted by the devil, or who were convinced that the world was about to come to an end. In short, there is little question that the human beings to whom the melancholia label was affixed often experienced great pain and despair.

It follows that 'experience' looms large over the history of melancholia, as it does over historical scholarship more broadly. A source of frustration for some historians and of fascination for others, experience is that slippery, perpetually unstable concept that can neither be pinned down nor ignored. The relationship between knowledge and experience is a particularly difficult, indeed often treacherous, space to navigate. When new knowledge and forms of classification are established, new facts are created. One way of understanding this process holds that psychiatric knowledge offers new ways of experiencing psychological phenomena, and that experience is subsequently fed back into the new categories, reinforcing these—producing what Ian Hacking has called a 'looping effect'.[60] While the culturally and historically contingent nature of experience has been convincingly demonstrated,[61] it remains a central, if contested, feature of the history of psychiatry, and the history of melancholia is no exception. The experiences of people diagnosed with melancholia lay beneath and informed the intellectual work that produced diagnostic language and, more broadly, psychiatric knowledge, but they are not the focus of this story. Not because they are not important, but because the object of scrutiny here is psychiatric knowledge: the aim is to understand how psychiatry creates its facts and truths. To the extent that patients feature in the present narrative, they do so primarily as descriptions and labels in textbooks, journal articles, asylum reports, and case notes.

This book takes classification to be a key event in the history of melancholia and depression, and of psychiatry more broadly. It has been a topic and source of much contention since the early years of the profession, and psychiatric categories have a significant, indeed sometimes life-changing, impact on the lives of individuals whose experiences are classified as mental disorders. To understand psychiatric knowledge, its role in care and treatment, and in shaping perceptions of selfhood, one must understand classification—how it is produced and applied, and the work it does in different contexts. Classification in psychiatry is primarily descriptive, and this has been the case since modern nosologies emerged in the nineteenth century. While physiology provided a useful framework for explaining disordered emotion, such models were of little practical use on asylum wards. They did not offer diagnostic tools to be deployed in determining the disease of a newly admitted patient. Instead, melancholia had to be identified and diagnosed according to a number of observable symptoms, primarily of the emotional kind. These could be deduced from communication with the patient, from enquiring into their actions prior to arriving in the asylum, and from observing the patient's demeanour, mode of speech, body language, motor function, and actions.

There was a dearth of home-grown British medical literature on insanity in the first half of the nineteenth century; no standard British nosology existed. Some physicians rejected melancholia as a diagnostic category, whereas others deployed it alongside other forms of chiefly emotional disorders, specifically monomania and moral insanity. However, in the second half of the nineteenth century melancholia was made increasingly coherent in British medical literature, in part though continuing uptake of German research. The disease picture that emerged was surprisingly consistent for a period when psychiatry was still an infant profession with few established norms and standards save for the legalities of incarceration and treatment. A physician who had read any of the major late nineteenth-century British textbooks on mental disease would know that the typical signs of melancholia were depressed mood, mental pain, despondency, despair, fear, delusions (often of a religious nature), refusal of food, inertia, restlessness, sleeplessness, and in some cases hallucinations, in particular hearing voices. Another key feature, which would become nearly as defining as the primary symptom of depressed mood, was the presence of suicidal tendencies. Melancholia was in many ways a broad medical concept, but it is misleading to dismiss the category, as one historian has done, as 'too vague and all-encompassing'.[62] It was a broad concept, but towards the end of the century, the disease picture was seen as relatively coherent, stable, and homogenous. The illness was often divided into a number of subcategories, but key symptoms were largely seen to apply across the board. Descriptions of melancholia were anything but vague—they were detailed and precise, both in published literature and in asylum records.

Nineteenth-century classification of affective insanity holds a marginal place in existing scholarship on melancholia and depression, despite the continued influence of nosologies and methods of classification developed in this period. German Berrios notes that the taxonomy of insanity underwent a profound shift in the modern period, which included the introduction of 'time' as a diagnostic feature. Importantly, he also notes that the emergence of descriptive psychopathology arose out of 'the failure of the anatomo-clinical model of mental disease which left alienists with mere symptom descriptions'.[63] He does not, however, address the other crucial development that emerged in response to the limits of anatomical models of mental disease: the appropriation of language and concepts from experimental physiology. As I show in subsequent chapters, these had a significant impact on how symptoms were interpreted, described, explained, and labelled. In this book, classification is understood as an historical event and a productive act. Melancholia was made (or re-made) in the nineteenth century as a modern, biomedical disease category. People who were diagnosed with melancholia were not incorrectly labelled; the act of diagnosing created melancholic patients, who in published material displayed a specific and largely consistent symptomatology. As will be seen in Chapter 6, however, the unity of this apparently coherent and delineated medical condition was achieved through the merging and flattening of a highly uneven and varied field of human experience through the use of standardised terminology and recording practices.

Before proceeding to tell this story, and bearing in mind the different concerns relating to melancholia and the history of psychiatry briefly outlined above, I want to emphasise what this book is not. It is not the history of an emotion. Neither is it a history of how people experienced melancholia in the nineteenth century. More broadly, it is not a social history of psychiatry or of the asylum as an institution. It is a history of a disease concept, specifically how this concept was reconfigured in nineteenth-century (primarily British) psychological medicine (later psychiatry). In this way, it is best understood as an intellectual history of psychiatric knowledge.[64] Statements are here taken to be historical acts with a productive force,[65] and clinical and administrative practices are taken to form part of the intellectual work that produced melancholia as a modern mood disorder. In mapping this process, the book draws on a range of sources, including psychiatric and medical textbooks, journal articles, legal records, lunacy commission directives, and asylum records, in particular statistical data and casebooks. In regard to the latter, Chapter 6 utilises records from several different asylums, each of which has its own particular history. Some of these institutions have been the focus of rich historical studies, which form part of an important and fascinating chapter in the history of madness and of medicine and society more widely. Here, however, asylum records are drawn upon for a specific purpose—to map how the melancholia diagnosis and its defining criteria were shaped and reified on the journey back and forth between case notes and published literature. Archival sources such as casebooks and diagnostic data sets are read as texts, part of a range of textual sources that together constitute what nineteenth-century psychiatrists said about melancholia and disordered mood at this time, and what knowledge was produced through these statements. To sum up, this book is the story of how melancholia was constituted as a specific type of illness in the nineteenth century: a modern mood disorder with a biomedical basis and a descriptive symptomatology.

STRUCTURE OF THE BOOK

The book begins in the early decades of the nineteenth century, when physiology was being established as the foundation of internal medicine. Chapter 2 maps the early appropriation of language and concepts from experimental physiology to explain mental phenomena. Through the works of early-to-mid-nineteenth-century physiologists and medical doctors schooled in the new science, the reader is introduced to the physiological origins of medico-psychological terms such as 'irritation', 'reflexion', and 'tone' that would be used to explain cerebral activity. These early writers provided the framework for the next generation of scientists who applied the findings of empirical research on sensory-motor action to the realm of ideas and emotion, and in doing so, established a new kind of mental science, physiological psychology. The chapter considers how Thomas Laycock and W.B. Carpenter, who had studied together in London, both created a model for mental reactivity, or psychological reflex action, that would form the framework for explaining disordered mood.

Chapter 3 picks up the historical trajectory of melancholia and affective insanity at a moment of significant change in perceptions of madness. Turn of the century asylum physicians and others treating the insane had increasingly favoured the new 'moral treatment', presented as a humanitarian and modern approach contrasted with older practices of restraint. This new approach not only transformed the treatment of the insane, but also ideas about what constituted insanity. The idea that one could be mad without being delusional was increasingly popularised in the first decades of the nineteenth century and provided an important philosophical foundation for the concept of disordered mood as a mental disease. The chapter traces the uptake of these ideas in mid-century British medical literature through the works of early influential physicians

J.C. Prichard and John Conolly. Finally, the chapter notes how mid-century British asylum physicians began to draw on physiology to explain disordered mood, and how melancholia was gradually reconfigured within this context.

Chapter 4 maps the establishment of a new, scientific model of mental disease in British psychological medicine, through the uptake of physiology as well as German psychiatry into mid-Victorian medical literature. In Germany, psychiatry was an established academic discipline by the 1860s, and a new generation of doctors promoted a strictly biological approach to mental disease. The chapter traces the conceptual history of disordered mood from Wilhelm Griesinger's early work on psychological reflex action, through his later psychiatric publications, through to Richard Krafft-Ebing's 1874 monograph on melancholia, in which it is presented as a distinct psychiatric category with a clear neurobiological foundation. The chapter then goes on to consider how Henry Maudsley successfully merged physiology and mental pathology in one of the century's most influential textbooks on mental disease, in which established a firm division between 'affective' and 'ideational' insanity. The development of this new approach to disordered mood is followed into the 1870s and 80s, where it was rapidly embraced by British asylum physicians across the country. Finally, melancholia is contrasted with neurasthenia, another nineteenth-century condition that was particularly popular in North America.

In Chapter 5 the story departs from internal medicine and turns instead to the administrative framework that was being constructed in Britain from the 1840s onward, where the creation of a national Lunacy Commission to oversee asylums produced a new bureaucracy of madness that sought to standardise diagnostic systems across the country. Asylum physicians were increasingly under pressure from lunacy commissioners to record a wide range of information about their patients, including symptoms and diagnoses, and compile such data into statistical tables and reports. Such numerical data was central to the standardisation of melancholia as a relatively stable and coherent diagnostic category with suicidality as a defining feature. The chapter goes on to show how the melancholia diagnosis coalesced around four distinct symptoms which became defining of the disease category in the last quarter of the century: mental pain, depression, suicidal tendencies, and religious delusions. We will see that these four keywords have remarkably different histories and that their emergence as defining symptoms of melancholia was the result of significant intellectual work coupled with new administrative practices as well as attempts to develop psychiatry as a medical profession and academic discipline.

Chapter 6 traces the processes of classification and diagnostics to the asylum ward. The casebooks of Edinburgh Royal Asylum form the focal point of the chapter, and are contrasted with records from other asylums. The chapter follows melancholia as it was reified through the circular and mutually constitutive relationship between asylum records and published material. Yet this relationship was also one characterised by tension and ambiguity. As narrative accounts of patients' mental states gave way to singular keywords, the description of symptoms appeared to become more precise and homogenous. The act of merging a range of expressions into descriptive key words facilitated more efficient recording of symptoms and presentation of cases in professional publications. At the same time, however, this practice changed what was recorded, producing new information about people. This chapter sheds light on the significant intellectual labour required to turn the chaos of human emotionality into neat medical categories.

Finally, the Conclusion briefly sketches out some of the shifts that began to occur at the turn of the century, in particular Emil Kraepelin's nosological division of insanity into dementia praecox and manic-depressive insanity, and Adolf Meyer's introduction of 'depression' as an illness category rather than a symptom of melancholia. These acts had significant consequences for the continued usage of the melancholia diagnosis, which rapidly declined in the twentieth century. The Conclusion places nineteenth-century melancholia in the context of twentieth- and twenty-first-century debates around mood disorders, descriptive psychopathology, and the ubiquity of clinical depression, asking how a critical historical approach to disordered mood can help us better understand—and critique—contemporary medical views on emotional distress. Finally, the Conclusion suggests some of the possible implications of attempts to revive biomedical melancholia as a diagnostic category in present psychiatry, and of attaching psychiatric labels to the emotional life of human beings.

Notes

1. Michel Foucault, *History of Madness* (London: Routledge, 2006 [1961]), 273.
2. Thomas S. Clouston, *Clinical Lectures on Mental Diseases* (London: J & A Churchill, 1883), 35.
3. David Healy, *The Antidepressant Era* (Cambridge, MA: Harvard University Press, 1997).
4. See for instance Allan V. Horwitz and Jerome C. Wakefield, *The Loss of Sadness: How Psychiatry Transformed Normal Sorrow into Depressive Disorder* (Oxford: Oxford University Press, 2007).
5. Brandon H. Hidaka, "Depression as a Disease of Modernity: Explanations for Increasing Prevalence," *Journal of Affective Disorders* 140 (2012): 211.
6. For a longer discussion of this approach in the context of the history of melancholia and depression, see Åsa Jansson, "Melancholia and Depression," *Oxford Research Encyclopedia of Psychology* (April 30, 2020), retrieved May 20, 2020, from https://oxfordre.com/psycho logy/view/10.1093/acrefore/9780190236557.001.0001/acrefore-978 0190236557-e-623.
7. The resurrection of melancholia was the subject of an interdisciplinary meeting in Copenhagen, the proceedings of which were subsequently published as a supplement issue of Acta Psychiatrica Scandinavica. *Acta Psychiatrica Scandinavica*, 115, Supplement 433 (2007). See also Michael A. Taylor and Max Fink, *Melancholia: The Diagnosis, Pathophysiology, and Treatment of Depressive Illness* (Cambridge: Cambridge University Press, 2006); Max Fink and Edward Shorter, *Endocrine Psychiatry: Solving the Riddle of Melancholia* (Oxford: Oxford University Press, 2010); Gordon Parker et al., "Issues for DSM-5: Whither Melancholia? The Case for Its Classification as a Distinct Mood Disorder," *American Journal of Psychiatry* 167, No. 7 (2010): 745–747.
8. Max Fink and Michael A. Taylor, "The Medical, Evidenced-Based Model for Psychiatric Syndromes: Return to a Classical Paradigm," *Acta Psychiatrica Scandinavica* 117 (2008): 82–83.
9. See esp. Stanley W. Jackson, *Melancholia and Depression: From Hippocratic Times to Modern Times* (New Haven and London: Yale University Press, 1986); Mikkel Borch-Jacobsen, *Making Minds and Madness: From Hysteria to Depression* (Cambridge: Cambridge University Press, 2009); Clark Lawlor, *From Melancholia to Prozac: A History of Depression* (Oxford: Oxford University Press, 2012). For a more nuanced approach, but which nonetheless comes down on the side of the continuity narrative, see Somogy Varga, "From Melancholia to Depression: Ideas on a Possible

Continuity," *Philosophy, Psychiatry, & Psychology* 20, No. 2 (2013): 141–155. For a critique of continuity narrative, see Jennifer Radden, "Is This Dame Melancholy? Equating Today's Depression and Past Melancholia," *Philosophy, Psychiatry, & Psychology* 10, No. 1 (2003): 37–52.

10. Max Fink and Michael A. Taylor, "Resurrecting Melancholia," *Acta Psychiatrica Scandinavica* 115, S. 433 (2007): 15.
11. L.S. Jacyna, "Somatic Theories of Mind and the Interests of Medicine in Britain, 1850–1879," *Medical History* 26 (1982): 237. Emphasis in original.
12. William F. Bynum, "The Nervous Patient in Eighteenth- and Nineteenth-Century Britain: The Psychiatric Origins of British Neurology," in *The Anatomy of Madness: Essays in the History of Psychiatry, Vol. I: People and Ideas*, eds. William F. Bynum, Roy Porter, and Michael Shepherd (London: Routledge, 1985), 90.
13. For psychiatric autopsies in nineteenth-century British psychiatry, see e.g. Jonathan Andrews, "Death and the Dead-House in the Victorian Asylum: Necroscopy versus Mourning at the Royal Edinburgh Asylum, c. 1832–1901," *History of Psychiatry* 23 (2012): 6–26; Jennifer Wallis, *Investigating the Body in the Victorian Asylum: Doctors, Patients, and Practices* (London: Palgrave Macmillan, 2017).
14. Clouston, *Clinical Lectures*, 37.
15. Kurt Danziger, "Mid-Nineteenth-Century British Psycho-Physiology: A Neglected Chapter in the History of Psychology," and Lorraine J. Daston, "The Theory of Will versus the Science of Mind," both in *The Problematic Science: Psychology in Nineteenth-Century Thought*, eds. William R. Woodward and Mitchell G. Ash (New York: Praeger, 1982); L.S. Jacyna, "The Physiology of Mind, the Unity of Nature, and the Moral Order in Victorian Thought," *British Journal for the History of Science* 14 (1981): 109–132, and "Somatic Theories of Mind"; Roger Smith, "Physiological Psychology and the Philosophy of Nature in Mid-Nineteenth Century Britain" (PhD diss., University of Cambridge, 1971).
16. Emily Martin's now classic essay offers an astute and important discussion of what happens when metaphorical (and value-laden) language eventually becomes reified and—seemingly—neutralised: Emily Martin, "The Egg and the Sperm: How Science Has Constructed a Romance Based on Stereotypical Male–Female Roles," *Signs* 16, No. 3 (1991): 485–501.
17. Craig Venter and Daniel Cohen, "The Century of Biology," *New Perspectives Quarterly* 21, No. 4 (2004): 73–77.

18. William Lawrence suggested this term in English following Gottfried Reinhold Treviranus' *Biologie* as the 'philosophy of living nature'. See William Lawrence, *Lectures on Physiology, Zoology, and the Natural History of Man: Delivered at the Royal College of Surgeons* (London: Benbow, 1822), 52. As Nikolas Rose suggests, however, the term is multivalent; 'there is no one biology in this "biological age".' Nikolas Rose, "The Human Sciences in a Biological Age," *Theory, Culture & Society* 30, No. 3 (2013): 5.

19. The *OED* traces 'biomedicine' and 'biomedical' to 1922 and 1921 respectively; the terms did not, however, gain widespread popularity until after WWII.

20. Adele E. Clarke, Janet K. Shim, Laura Mamo, Jennifer R. Fosket, and Jennifer R. Fishman, "Biomedicalization: Technoscientific Transformations of Health, Illness and U.S. Biomedicine," *American Sociological Review* 68 (2003): 162.

21. E.g. Janet Oppenheim, *'Shattered Nerves': Doctors, Patients, and Depression in Victorian England* (Oxford: Oxford University Press, 1991); Anita Guerrini, *Depression and Obesity in the Enlightenment: The Life and Times of George Cheyne* (Norman: University of Oklahoma Press, 2000); Lawlor, *From Melancholia to Prozac*; Margaret Sorbie Thompson, "The Mad, the Bad, and the Sad: Psychiatric Care in the Royal Edinburgh Asylum (Morningside), 1813–1894" (PhD diss., Boston University, 1984).

22. E.g. George Cheyne, *An Essay of Health and Long Life*, 2nd ed. (London: George Strahan, 1725), 100; George Berkeley, "Three Dialogues between Hylas and Philonous," in *The Works of George Berkeley, Vol. II: Philosophical Works*, ed. Alexander Campbell (Oxford: Clarendon Press, 1901), 98; David Hume, *Essays, Moral and Political* (Edinburgh: R. Fleming & A. Alison, 1741), 145.

23. German E. Berrios, "Melancholia and Depression during the Nineteenth Century: A Conceptual History," *British Journal of Psychiatry* 153 (1988): 298–304; Judith Misbach and Henderikus J. Stam, "Medicalizing Melancholia: Exploring Profiles of Psychiatric Professionalization," *Journal of the History of the Behavioral Sciences* 42, No. 1 (2006): 41–59.

24. For a critique of the cultural universality of modern depression from an anthropological perspective, see Sushrut Jadhav, "The Cultural Origins of Western Depression," *International Journal of Social Psychiatry* 42 (1996): 269–286.

25. John C. Bucknill and Daniel Hack Tuke, *A Manual of Psychological Medicine*, 4th ed. (London: J & A Churchill, 1879), 215; Roy Porter, *The Greatest Benefit to Mankind: A Medical History of Humanity* (New York and London: W. W. Norton, 1997), 56–60.

26. Angus Gowland, "The Problem of Early Modern Melancholy," *Past and Present* 191 (2006): 86. See also Matthew Bell, *Melancholia: The Western Malady* (Cambridge: Cambridge University Press, 2014); Jennifer Radden, "Introduction," in *The Nature of Melancholy: From Aristotle to Kristeva*, ed. Jennifer Radden (New York: Oxford University Press 2000); Erin Sullivan, *Beyond Melancholy: Sadness and Selfhood in Renaissance Britain* (Oxford: Oxford University Press, 2016); Wolf Lepenies, *Melancholy and Society* (Cambridge, MA: Harvard University Press, 1992).

27. With the gradual decline in popularity of the humoural model, other explanations for melancholia emerged. For instance, Thomas Willis suggested in the seventeenth century that 'we cannot here yield, to what some Physicians affirm, that Melancholy doth arise from a Melancholick humor', rather, 'it ought to be affirmed, that this distemper doth sometimes first begin from the Brain, and the Soul dwelling within it.' Thomas Willis, *Two Discourses Concerning the Soul of Brutes* (London: Thomas Dring, 1683), 192.

28. Jeremy Schmidt, "Melancholy and the Therapeutic Language of Moral Philosophy in Seventeenth-Century Thought," *Journal of the History of Ideas* 65, No. 4 (2004): 583; Jackson, *Melancholia and Depression*, 29; Roy Porter, "Mood Disorders: Social Section," in *A History of Clinical Psychiatry, the Origin and History of Psychiatric Disorders*, eds. German E. Berrios and Roy Porter (London: Athlone Press, 1995), 409. Berrios refers to earlier (pre-modern) forms of melancholia as 'a rag-bag of insanity states'. German E. Berrios, "Mood Disorders: Clinical Section," in *A History of Clinical Psychiatry*, 385. See also Berrios, "Melancholia and Depression," 298.

29. Gowland, "Early Modern Melancholy," 87–88.

30. Karin Johannisson, *Melankoliska rum: om ångest, leda och sårbarhet i förfluten tid och nutid* (Stockholm: Bonniers, 2009), 76.

31. Reinhard Kuhn, *The Demon of Noontide: Ennui in Western Literature* (Princeton, NJ: Princeton University Press, 1976), 39–64.

32. Johannisson, *Melankoliska rum*, 42–43. See also e.g. Willis, *Soul of Brutes*, 188: '[S]ome have believed themselves to be Dogs or Wolves, and have imitated their ways and kind by barking or howling; others have thought themselves dead, desiring presently to be buried; others imagining that their bodies were made of glass, were afraid to be touched lest they should be broke to pieces.' Cf. '*mania lupina*', in where 'sufferers [were] displaying strongly negative aspects of wolfish behaviour: they are wild, riotous and can only be placated with great difficulty using shackles.' Nadine Metzger, "Battling Demons with Medical Authority: Werewolves, Physicians, and Rationalization," *History of Psychiatry* 24, No. 3 (2013): 346.

33. See e.g. George Cheyne, *The English Malady, or, a Treatise of Nervous Diseases of All Kinds, as Spleen, Vapour, Lowness of Spirits, Hypochondriacal or Hysterical Distempers* (London: George Strahan, 1733).

34. George Beard, *A Practical Treatise on Nervous Exhaustion (Neurasthenia), Its Symptoms, Nature, Sequences, Treatment* (New York: William Wood, 1880).

35. Notable works include: Bell, *Melancholia*; Angus Gowland, *The Worlds of Renaissance Melancholy: Robert Burton in Context* (Cambridge: Cambridge University Press, 2006); Johannisson, *Melankoliska rum*; Lawlor, *From Melancholia to Prozac*; Darian Leader, *The New Black: Mourning, Melancholia and Depression* (London: Hamish Hamilton, 2008); Lepenies, *Melancholy and Society*; Radden, *The Nature of Melancholy*; Sullivan, *Beyond Melancholy*.

36. Johannisson, *Melankoliska rum*, 13. This question has also been posed by Barbara Rosenwein, who uses the term 'emotional communities' to describe the different ways in which emotions have been experienced in different times and cultures. Barbara H. Rosenwein, "Worrying about Emotions in History," *American Historical Review* 107, No. 3 (2002): 821–845.

37. David Walker and Anita O'Connell give significant weight to both perspectives, suggesting that pre-modern descriptions of low mood 'certainly [appear] to match' DSM criteria for depression, but that 'because those specific frameworks, no longer exist … earlier forms 'of melancholy cannot be said to be the same as depression.' David Walker and Anita O'Connell, "Introduction," in *Depression and Melancholy, 1660–1800, Vol 1: General Introduction & Religious Writings*, eds. Leigh Wetherall Dickson, Allan Ingram, David Walker, and Anita O'Connell (London: Pickering & Chatto, 2012).

38. Jackson, *Melancholia and Depression*, ix.

39. The same argument has been made previously by Allan Horwitz and Jerome Wakefield in their critical analysis of the creation of Major Depressive Disorder. It is worth noting that Robert Spitzer, the head of the *DSM-III* task force who was a key target of Horwitz and Wakefield's critique, took on board some of their criticisms, and even wrote a preface to their book where he noted that 'Dr. Wakefield has critiqued my efforts in ways that I have largely become convinced are valid'. Robert Spitzer, "Preface," in Horwitz and Wakefield, *The Loss of Sadness*, viii.

40. Edward Shorter, "The Doctrine of the Two Depressions in Historical Perspective," *Acta Psychiatrica Scandinavica* 115, S433 (2007): 5–13. Falling somewhere between a continuity perspective and one that emphasises historical shifts, George Rousseau perceives the distinction between two forms of depression to be chiefly historical, in the form of 'a premedicalized category (*melancholia*) and a post-medicalized (*depression*).'

Nevertheless, he holds that 'the older version contained a sufficient quantity of the characteristics of the newer to permit the conceptualization of a "history of depression" as if it had been a single, continuous category.' George Rousseau, "Depression's Forgotten Genealogy: Notes towards a History of Depression," *History of Psychiatry* 11 (2000): 74.

41. Misbach and Stam, "Medicalizing Melancholia," 44–45.

42. Berrios, "Melancholia and Depression," 300–301.

43. Bell, *Melancholia*, 3.

44. William F. Bynum and Michael Neve, "Hamlet on the Couch," in *The Anatomy of Madness: Essays in the History of Psychiatry, Vol. I: People and Ideas*, eds. William F. Bynum, Roy Porter, and Michael Shepherd (London: Routledge, 1985), 290.

45. See for instance Chapter 17 of Ian Hacking's *Rewriting the Soul* ('An indeterminacy in the past'), and the subsequent debate that played out on the pages of the *History of the Human Sciences*, which has become known as the 'Chapter 17 debate': Wes Sharrock and Ivan Leudar, "Indeterminacy in the Past?" *History of the Human Sciences* 15, No. 3 (2002): 95–115; Steve Fuller, "Making Up the Past: a Response to Sharrock and Leudar," *History of the Human Sciences* 15, No. 4 (2002): 115–123; Ian Hacking, "Indeterminacy in the Past: On the Recent Discussion of Chapter 17 of Rewriting the Soul," *History of the Human Sciences* 16, No. 2 (2003): 117–124; Kevin McMillan, "Under a Redescription," *History of the Human Sciences* 16, No. 2 (2003): 129–150. See also Ian Hacking, *Rewriting the Soul: Multiple Personality and the Sciences of Memory* (Princeton, NJ: Princeton University Press, 1995).

46. Jerome Kroll and Bernard Bachrach, *The Mystic Mind: The Psychology of Medieval Mystics and Ascetics* (New York: Routledge, 2005), 25–28.

47. George Cheyne, for instance, an eighteenth-century physician who produced several comprehensive texts on the 'nervous disorders' of his time, and who also wrote publicly on his own struggles with these, has been described as suffering from 'depression' and 'obesity'. Guerrini, *Depression and Obesity*.

48. Bell, *Melancholia*, 8. See also Dominic Murphy, *Psychiatry in the Scientific Image* (Cambridge, MA: MIT Press, 2006).

49. My approach to the history of disease concepts and of the emotions is indebted to a number of writers, from history, sociology, anthropology, literature, and the philosophy of science. Of particular significance are: Georges Canguilhem, *The Normal and the Pathological* (New York: Zone Books, 1989); Thomas Dixon, *From Passions to Emotions: The Creation of a Secular Psychological Category* (Cambridge: Cambridge University Press, 2003); Michel Foucault, *Psychiatric Power: Lectures at the Collège de France, 1973–74* (Basingstoke: Palgrave Macmillan, 2006), *The Archaeology of Knowledge* (London and New York: Routledge, 2002 [1969]),

and *History of Madness*; Ian Hacking, "Making Up People," reprinted in *Beyond the Body Proper: Reading the Anthropology of Material Life*, eds. Margaret Lock and Judith Farquhar (Durham: Duke University Press, 2007), and "The Looping Effects of Human Kinds," in *Causal Cognition: A Multidisciplinary Debate*, eds. Dan Sperber, David Premack, and Ann James Premack (Oxford: Clarendon Press, 1995); Annemarie Mol, *The Body Multiple: Ontology in Medical Practice* (Durham: Duke University Press, 2002); Adrian Wilson, "On the History of Disease-Concepts: The Case of Pleurisy," *History of Science* 38, No. 3 (2000): 304–305; Allan Young, *The Harmony of Illusions: Inventing Post-Traumatic Stress Disorder* (Princeton, NJ: Princeton University Press, 1995).

50. Foucault, *Psychiatric Power*, 266.

51. E.g. Andrew Scull, *The Most Solitary of Afflictions: Madness and Society in Britain 1700–1900* (New Haven: Yale University Press, 1993); Eric J. Engstrom, *Clinical Psychiatry in Imperial Germany: A History of Psychiatric Practice* (Ithaca, NY: Cornell University Press, 2004); Misbach and Stam, "Medicalizing Melancholia".

52. See for instance Foucault, *Psychiatric Power* and *History of Madness*; Marcel Gauchet and Gladys Swain, *Madness and Democracy: The Modern Psychiatric Universe* (Princeton, NJ: Princeton University Press, 1999); Andrew Scull, *The Insanity of Place, the Place of Insanity: Essays on the History of Psychiatry* (London: Routledge, 2006).

53. See for instance Ann Goldberg, *Sex, Religion and the Making of Modern Madness: The Eberbach Asylum and German Society, 1815–1849* (Oxford: Oxford University Press, 1999); and on recovering the patient's perspective in the history of medicine more generally, see Roy Porter, "The Patient's View: Doing Medical History from Below," *Theory and Society* 14, No. 2 (1985): 175–198.

54. A good starting point for anyone wishing to explore the field is: Andrew Scull, ed., *Madhouses, Mad-Doctors, and Madmen: The Social History of Psychiatry in the Victorian Era* (Philadelphia: University of Pennsylvania Press, 1981).

55. Joseph Melling and Bill Forsythe, *The Politics of Madness: The State, Insanity, and Society in England, 1845–1914* (London: Routledge, 2006).

56. The central role of asylum practices in the production of psychiatric and medical knowledge has increasingly become the focus of historical interrogation in recent years. Of particular importance is Sarah Chaney's book on the history of self-harm, which draws on records from Bethlem, as well as Jennifer Wallis' study shedding light of the significance of the body in the production of psychiatric knowledge, which centres on the Wakefield asylum. Both authors skilfully map the intellectual work that took place in these institutions in the processes of diagnosis, treatment, and (in the case of Wallis) post-mortem examinations. Sarah Chaney, *Psyche on the Skin: A*

History of Self-Harm (London: Reaktion Books, 2017), Chapter 2; Wallis, *Investigating the Body in the Victorian Asylum*.

57. The use of statistics has also played a significant role in the formation and diagnosis of non-psychological disease concepts. See e.g. Lloyd G. Stevenson, "Exemplary Disease: The Typhoid Pattern," *Journal of the History of Medicine and Allied Sciences* 37, No. 4 (1982): 159–181.

58. An important exception is Trevor Turner's study of the records of Ticehurst in Sussex (which are briefly drawn upon in Chapter 6). Trevor Turner, *A Diagnostic Analysis of the Casebooks of Ticehurst House Asylum, 1845–1890* (Cambridge: Cambridge University Press, 1992).

59. Melling and Forsythe, *The Politics of Madness*, 189.

60. In a critical interrogation of Hacking's approach, Chris Millard importantly reminds us that the tools we use to critique the presumed universality of existing concepts are themselves products of specific historical contexts. In other words, we must be aware of 'the boundedness and historical specificity of the "malleable humanity"'. Chris Millard, "Concepts, Diagnosis and the History of Medicine: Historicising Ian Hacking and Munchausen Syndrome," *Social History of Medicine* 30, No. 3 (2017): 589.

61. Joan Wallach Scott, "The Evidence of Experience," *Critical Inquiry* 17, No. 4 (1991): 773–797.

62. Goldberg, *Sex, Religion and the Making of Modern Madness*, 5.

63. Berrios, *The History of Mental Symptoms*, 302.

64. My approach to the history of ideas is in particular indebted to Gadamer. See Hans-Georg Gadamer, *Truth and Method* (New York: Continuum, 2003 [1960]) and "The Problem of Historical Consciousness," in *Interpretive Social Science: A Reader*, eds. Paul Rabinow and William M. Sullivan (Berkeley: University of California Press, 1979).

65. I take my cue here from J.L. Austin and Judith Butler. J.L. Austin, *How to Do Things with Words* (Oxford: Clarendon Press, 1962), esp. pp. 6–8, 101–108, 120–122; Judith Butler, *Excitable Speech: A Politics of the Performative* (New York: Routledge, 1997).

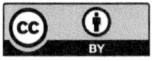

CHAPTER 2

The Scientific Foundation of Disordered Mood

The scalpel and microscope will alike fail; the meditations of metaphysicians will come to nought; the disease will remain in its status quo, a phantom and a fear. To the pure doctrine of physiology, we must look for the first glimpse of truth, and by the close application of its principles shall we soonest find the path; while without its help in the study of cerebral disease we shall never attain our end.[1]

J. Hawkes (1855)

In a paper read before the British Association for the Advancement of Science in 1844, physiologist Thomas Laycock described to his audience the case of a young boy who suffered from hydrophobia (a fear of water). He quoted a Mr. Thornhill who had originally published the case in the *Medical Gazette*:

On suggesting that he should swallow a little water, [the boy] seemed to be frightened, and began to cry out. He turned suddenly in bed, and was simultaneously seized with a momentary clonic spasm of the trunk, greatly resembling emprosthotonos [a spasm in which the head and feet meet and the back is arched]; however, by kindly encouraging him, he soon manifested a willingness to accede my wish, but the sound of the water as it was poured into a teacup, again brought on a similar convulsive action.[2]

© The Author(s) 2021
Å Jansson, *From Melancholia to Depression,*
Mental Health in Historical Perspective,
https://doi.org/10.1007/978-3-030-54802-5_2

The boy's reaction showed, Laycock argued, that 'the idea of water excites convulsion', proving his thesis that the kind of reflexive model normally reserved for sensory-motor activity also applied to the brain and the mind. In other words, just like involuntary movement could be triggered by sensory stimuli, an abstract idea could act as a trigger for involuntary emotion as well as motor action. While this was at the time a radical idea, it would become one of the most influential and durable psychological principles of the modern period. But how did Laycock arrive at his argument? And what were the implications of such a model of mental operations? This chapter traces the origins of psychological reflex action, the scientific principle that formed the basis for the idea of disordered mood as a medical concept. It begins in the early years of the nineteenth century, when experimental physiology was taking Europe by storm. British scientists such as Marshall Hall and Charles Bell were attempting to describe the functions of the spinal nerves while navigating the gradual and equivocal shift from older ideas about 'sympathy' to a modern framework for physical reactivity. Physiology, the new science of the body with its growing catalogue of empirical evidence, was a goldmine for physicians trying to make sense of and treat the maladies of the mind, and it was rapidly absorbed into medical textbooks for students and practitioners.

The first part of the chapter is concerned with the physiological language of internal medicine from where Laycock drew the analogies used to explain psychological reflexion and, subsequently, disordered emotion. The function of analogous language is central to the emergence of a biomedical language of emotion, and plays a key role in the story of nineteenth-century melancholia more widely. A number of the words used to describe features of melancholia, internal and external, were deployed both as literal descriptions of cerebral (and thus psychological) events, and as analogous to physical processes elsewhere in the body. Moreover, older theories often converged with the new, such as in the work of British physiologist W.B. Carpenter, who embraced a biological reflex model for some mental operations, while insisting on retaining a higher faculty independent from somatic automatism. In sum, biomedical theories of emotion were, at this time, new, fragmented, unsteady, conflicting, and constantly evolving. Nevertheless, within the emerging framework of what became known as physiological psychology, emotion was gradually constituted as a physiological process and a biomedical object of study. As will be seen in later chapters, melancholia was subsequently reconfigured along these new biomedical lines.

REFLEX ACTION, AUTOMATISM, AND EMOTION IN MEDICAL SCIENCE

The significant epistemological shifts that occurred in the first decades of the nineteenth century in terms of both scientific and lay perceptions of the natural world and the animal body have been thoroughly explored elsewhere.[3] What should be noted here is that the physiology of disordered emotion was to a large extent premised upon a belief that the mind could be explained as a manifestation of cerebral activity. Within the wider context of the rise of scientific medicine and secular psychology such beliefs made sense to a vast number of physicians. At the same time, however, materialist conceptions of the relationship between body, brain, mind, and soul were contentious and contested both within and outside scientific communities. For some medical scientists, such as Laycock, subscribing to a physiological model of cerebral activity meant the rejection of a higher, abstract intellect, but for others, most notably Laycock's acquaintance and intellectual rival Carpenter, a separation between soma and psyche was to some extent maintained. There was, as Roger Smith has suggested, 'nothing inevitable about these intellectual developments'.[4] The mind–body problem and the place of humans in the world were questions that pushed at both old and new boundaries of epistemology during the nineteenth century, and there was no clear or simple shift from the Christian to the secular or from the philosophical to the scientific. Rather, 'language often left unresolved a choice between new or old, between a concern with human culture or human science, between a religious or a secular world view.[5]

Nevertheless, physiological experiments performed on frogs and other animals in order to infer knowledge about the human nervous system were premised upon a belief that human beings were inherently part of the animal world and subject to the laws of nature. While humans held a hierarchically superior position in this world, experimental physiology as a path to knowledge about the human body made sense because human beings were perceived as having sufficient shared characteristics with other animals. This did not, however, mean that scientists rejected providence or a higher soul. When physicians began to speak about ideas and emotion as automated physiological processes this was for many a controversial move. Both within and beyond scientific communities physiologically anchored theories of mind met with objections from Christian writers. Thomas Dixon notes that reactions among Christian thinkers were far from unified; nonetheless, a shared point of antagonism between many of them was that the new physiological psychology left little or no room for a higher, abstract soul.[6] The idea of emotion as a reflexive, automated function was possible within a system of thought that took emotion to be a bodily and often also a *cerebral* process.[7] This latter point constituted an important division between physicians who believed in different models of psychological reflexion. The kind of model of involuntary reaction of emotion and ideas in conjunction that formed the basis for biomedical theories of melancholia generally held emotion to be a cerebral activity rather than a reaction occurring in a lower part of the nervous system. The significance of this distinction is illustrated below in the contrast between the psycho-physiological theories offered by Thomas Laycock and William Benjamin Carpenter.

Viewed as a psychological reaction, 'emotion' would in one sense become a broader category than the traditional 'passions', 'sentiments', and 'appetites'. As a secular, psychological category, 'emotion' would gradually replace such older terms anchored in a theistic language and view of the body–mind relationship. At the same time, however, emotion as understood within physiological psychology and psychological medicine was a narrow category, in that it was perceived as a process, or event, contained within the human nervous system.[8] This way of explaining the mental life of humans did not mesh comfortably with the possibility of an intellect belonging to a higher soul and capable of disciplining the lower animal appetites. However, as Smith has noted, the new scientific discourse about mind and body remained steeped in moral argument.[9] Indeed, as the century wore on a person's *im*morality became an increasingly biological feature, permanently imprinted on degenerate brains and bodies.[10]

THE REFLEX CONCEPT

The theory of reflexive action was a chief preoccupation of European physiologists early in the century and formed the basis of and rationale for numerous experiments on living animal bodies. Ruth Leys has referred to the reflex concept as espoused by nineteenth-century experimental scientists as 'one of the most influential explanatory principles in the history of the medical, biological, and psychological sciences', noting that 'it has played a major role in the rise of psychology as an experimental science'.[11] Smith and L.S. Jacyna have both drawn attention to the role of the reflex in the development of nineteenth-century British psychopathology.[12] Building on existing historical work in this vein, the emphasis here is on how the reflex model facilitated the creation of disordered mood as a medical concept, a concept that was foundational to melancholia as a modern biomedical mental disease. This transfer of knowledge from neurology and nervous physiology to psychology and psychiatry was neither inevitable nor straightforward, and, as is demonstrated below and in Chapter 4, a significant amount of intellectual labour was required to bring it about.

A driving force behind physiological research in the nineteenth century was the objective of 'knowing the body', and with it the brain. Roger Cooter has observed that the knowledge produced through such research had little practical use for ordinary people, the way earlier medical self-help manuals and recipe books had had. Yet this nascent science held the power to reveal 'what was hitherto a mystery for most people, the internal operations of their bodies.'[13] For scientists who believed that the production of ideas and emotions was the result of cerebral activity, knowing the body also meant knowing the mind. As suggested above, experiments on living animal bodies occurred within a belief system about the natural world without which it would not make sense to conduct such experiments in the first place. In this context, the nervous system was conceptualised and visualised along certain lines, it was discussed in terms of 'reactions', 'reflexes', 'sensation', 'irritation', stimulus', 'tone', and 'motion'.

While 'reflex' came to mean something quite specific in medico-scientific literature in the mid-to-late nineteenth century, the idea of reflexive action as something occurring inside the human body was not the invention of experimental physiologists. Any attempt to trace the origins of the reflex concept beyond the modern period must, however, be carried out with the same kind of historical and contextual sensitivity as is called for when comparing ancient, medieval, and early modern writings on melancholia with nineteenth-century literature. Historians (and nineteenth-century scientists) have offered different views on the history of the modern sensory-motor reflex. The invention of the concept has been attributed to Descartes,[14] whereas others have highlighted British physician Marshall Hall as one of the key figures in its creation.[15] Ruth Leys agrees that Hall's theory of the 'reflex arc' was central to modern ideas about involuntary reflexive action, but she cautions historians against perceiving the reflex as having 'developed in a linear or incremental fashion towards the present'.[16] Hall's theory of reflexive action was, she suggests, equally a rearticulation of older ideas about 'sympathy'; moreover, it was purely 'mechanistic', almost in a Cartesian sense. For Hall, '[t]he central nervous system was subject to the laws of the reflex as high as the medulla but no higher: above the cord was the entirely different cerebral system, the seat of the immortal soul'.[17] Hall's conception importantly allowed for volition as a faculty independent from and higher than reactions anchored in the body. In this way, it followed along the lines of older, broadly Christian beliefs, which held that the higher faculties were able to exert control over the lower ones (such as 'animal passions').[18]

Much of the language that came to be used to speak about emotion was metaphorical in its origins. While we may, as historians have done, speak about the reflex having been 'extended' to the realm of ideas and emotion, such a narrative suggests a progressive, indeed an almost teleological, development. Nineteenth-century scientists did not simply follow a path of step-by-step discovery. The acts and events that create scientific objects are never simple and uncontested, and the creation of psychological reflexion, and of disordered emotion, was a particularly imaginative endeavour. A new generation of scientists was keen to use novel empirical research to try to make sense of that which had perplexed and mystified European philosophers since antiquity—what is it that makes humans think, feel, act, and react? An area of inquiry that used to belong chiefly to philosophy was increasingly being staked out by medical scientists through the appropriation of medical language from the realm of the physical to that of the psychological. Concepts that have solid and naturalised meanings in psychology and psychiatry today began their journey as metaphors borrowed from internal medicine.

IRRITATION AND MORBID SENSIBILITY: FROM INTERNAL TO PSYCHOLOGICAL MEDICINE

As British writers themselves noted, most of the cutting-edge research in the area of experimental physiology was being carried out on the continent. However, home-grown publications were not entirely absent, and a handful of early Victorian authorities on the subject were emerging in the 1830s and 40s. Charles Bell and Marshall Hall were both important champions of neurophysiological theories on the continent as well as in Britain, and their work has been considered in detail by historians.

However, other less prominent writers also had a significant impact on the development of physiological psychology in Britain, and an even greater influence on the emerging concept of disordered mood. Of particular significance in this regard was Archibald Billing's popular *First Principles of Medicine*, published in several editions between the 1830s and the 1860s and widely consulted and cited by British physicians with an interest in the brain and the mind. Billing, physician, lecturer and clinical instructor at the London Hospital in Whitechapel,[19] eagerly emphasised his own role in the establishment of physiological ideas about cerebral activity, alongside some of his more famous peers.[20]

Billing's textbook underwent several revisions, but his approach to nervous action was strictly somatic from the outset. He suggested that all nervous function was best understood as analogous to electricity, and held that this may be more than an analogy, since the application of an electric current to the nerves would prompt muscle contraction (something which scientists had noted since the seventeenth century). Billing situated his treatise within the framework of experimental physiology, drawing indirectly upon experiments performed on living animals, particularly frogs, where surgically exposed nerves were subjected to electric currents intended to produce reflexive movement. In a presentation of different ways in which various bodily reactions simulated electricity, Billing also suggested as an example '[v]olition being conducted along the nerves with a speed equal only to electricity'.[21] In this way, the will was conceptualised as a physiological process; no distinction was made between involuntary reaction as somatic and voluntary action as mental.

Two things are important to note about Billing's work. First of all, his physiological model was a fusion of old and new language and concepts. Billing's illustration of nerve force bore evident resemblance to eighteenth-century natural philosophy, and ideas about 'irritation' as a trigger of nervous function looks superficially similar to von Haller's concept of 'irritability' put forward in the 1750s and which explained involuntary muscular reaction in response to stimuli. For Haller, however, 'the power of contraction resided in the muscle itself' and was the result of a 'nerve force' or *vis nervosa*.[22] This illustrates the argument made above, that while much early modern terminology was slow to disappear, similarity in language should not be mistaken for conceptual sameness. Secondly, we should not take his statement above to mean that Billing perceived volition as a reflexive act. He circumvented the problem of an independent will in a biological framework by suggesting that sensation, action, and reaction in the human body were carried along two different sets of nerves—voluntary and involuntary.[23] Despite this attempt to keep the will intact, we can note the possible consequences of Billing's argument. He made it clear to his readers that '[a]ll organic action is contraction, produced by nervous influence'.[24] This would appear to suggest that Billing held all mental activity to be a manifestation of such contraction; however, his somatic model of nervous activity did not extend to intellectual life. In other words, while volition was transmitted along nerve paths, it was not an automated somatic reaction. Not only did Billing perceive a separation between bodily activity and the mental faculties; the detailed study of 'the properties and processes' of the human body was ultimately a revelation of 'the omniscience of the Deity'. The body was, in the end, merely a 'structure' that 'the Soul' was 'destined to inhabit for but a short space of time'.[25]

In *First Principles of Medicine* we find a number of medical concepts that would become foundational to physiological theories of mental disease. Two of these are particularly important for our present enquiry: 'irritation' and 'morbid sensibility'. Billing used the latter to describe 'that state of the nerves or central organs which renders them more susceptible to impressions than natural'.[26] Billing explained the occurrence of such sensibility in different organs through the application of 'the reflex theory'. The inherent sensibility of nerves would render these susceptible to 'irritation', which in turn could produce morbid sensibility:

> If, therefore, certain diseased states, unaccompanied by pain, termed 'irritation' (which term can properly be applied only to whatever is the *cause* of the morbid sensibility), exist in a part of which the spinal cord takes cognizance, and which are indicated by subsequent production of abnormal muscular contractions, &c. in distant parts of the body, it follows that the spinal cord has become *sensible* of that diseased state, that is, has participated in the morbid sensibility, although the *brain* has not been informed of it.[27]

The idea of 'irritation' of the nerves causing an organ to become morbidly sensitive would become central to the kind of physiological explanation for disordered emotion offered by later writers. As will be seen below, it is important to note that Billing perceived this process as happening *without* cerebral involvement. By this he not only meant that the mind was not aware of it, but also that it was a reactive process that did not reach the brain hemispheres. In this way, Billing was consistent with standard medical opinion at the time in that he did not deviate from the distinction made by Hall and others between voluntary and involuntary action where the latter was somatic and the former cerebral or even outside of the body completely. In other words, involuntary action could only occur without cerebral involvement, as a reaction triggered below the brain, no further up than the medulla. It was a separation that was physical in its description, but of which the consequences were also psychological. However, as shall be seen in a moment, when scientists extrapolated such concepts to speak about ideas and emotion, a framework was created whereby involuntary reaction could occur in the brain but still without conscious awareness.

Billing went on to describe precisely how disease would arise from the state of irritation, suggesting that '[i]f the nerves of *sensation* be rendered morbidly sensitive, pain is produced by common occurrences which ought not to affect them, such as pressure either from external things, or even of the surrounding parts'.[28] This metaphor would above all become key to explaining biomedical melancholia; indeed one may go so far as to say that it formed the rationale for melancholia as a disorder. The idea of how a morbid reaction to normal impressions could occur would become part of standard descriptions of melancholia as a disease in which ordinary impressions that would trigger no emotional reaction in a healthy mind would produce 'mental pain' and 'depression'.[29] Similar models were offered by other contemporaneous British writers who, like Billing, referred much of the current knowledge on the anatomy and physiology of the nerves to Bell and Magendie. A work that received particular interest among mid-century medical psychologists was Samuel Solly's *The Human Brain*, first published in 1836 with an updated second edition a decade later. Solly's book was to a large extent an account and discussion of recent French research. The first edition was also chiefly concerned with the anatomy and physiology of animal brains—i.e. data directly derived from empirical research—with some extrapolations regarding the human brain.[30] Overall, two recurrent themes in particular should be noted in regard to British medico-scientific literature on the physiology of the nervous system prior to the 1840s: the idea that persistent 'irritation' of the nerves caused them to become more sensitive and prone to morbidity, and, a model of involuntary reflexive action that did not include the cerebral hemispheres in such activity.

FROM SENSORY-MOTOR REFLEX
TO PSYCHOLOGICAL AUTOMATISM

While Billing and Solly's frameworks were later taken up in and adapted to psychological medicine by the next generation of British physicians, in the early decades of British mental science the impact of work produced by continental writers was at least as substantial, if not more so. Prussian physiologist Johannes Müller's *Elements of Physiology*[31] navigated territory that Billing and many other contemporary physiologists had not ventured into. Müller was curious about the psychological implications of physiological research and attempted to draw parallels between the human psyche and sensory-motor experiments performed on animals. His work contains the beginnings of the kind of analogous transfer of concepts that would form the core of later theories about affective insanity. Müller's *Elements* provided mid-century physicians with tools allowing them to hypothesise about psychological (and thus emotional) reflexive action.

Müller, who trained rising stars such as Hermann von Helmholtz and Emil du Bois-Reymond, was appointed to the first German chair of physiology in 1833,[32] the same year as the first volume of his *Elements of Physiology* was published. This work drew upon experiments performed by Müller himself as well as data derived from other people's research, and a substantial chunk of the book was devoted to the workings of the nervous system, including the brain and the mind. For many early nineteenth-century German scientists, their convictions about the place of human beings as part of the animal kingdom and natural world were rooted in *Naturphilosophie*, generally regarded as belonging to Romanticism and, from a scientific point of view, somewhat pre-modern. However, as Jutta Schickore has suggested, these beliefs had much in common with later, post-Darwinian explanatory frameworks. In particular, the unity of 'Man' and nature is important in this regard, and philosophical ideas within this early tradition had an impact on scientific endeavours later on.[33] One of the most influential explanations of human ability to acquire knowledge about nature arising from *Naturphilosophie* came from Friedrich Schelling, who argued that 'we are able to have knowledge about the natural world because nature and the human subject are essentially the same'.[34] Müller came out of this tradition, but largely rejected Schelling's views. His own beliefs were complex, however, not least because he was a prolific researcher who carried out work within a vast number of different areas of physiology. Nevertheless, Schickore suggests that he was in the first instance concerned with 'the overall problem of how living things could be *experienced*'.[35] This perspective was important for how a new generation of scientists in the German-speaking areas approached their work. While for many laboratory scientists empirical research continued to be carried out within a loose framework of older philosophical and spiritual beliefs about the world, 'a new accent on academic, original research came together with an explicit preference for experience over speculation'.[36]

For Müller, emotion was a manifestation of nervous action; a physiological process of the interconnected brain-body system. Perhaps seeking to distance himself from the populist science of phrenology, he remarked that '[t]here are no data for either proving or refuting the hypothesis that the passions have their seat of action in a particular part of the brain'. He went on to emphasise the ability of emotion to trigger peripheral bodily reactions:

> The exciting passions give rise to spasms, and frequently even to convulsive motions affecting the muscles supplied by the respiratory and facial nerves. Not only are the features distorted, but the actions of the respiratory muscles are so changed as to produce the movements of crying, sighing, and sobbing. Any passion of whatever nature, if of sufficient intensity, may give rise to crying and sobbing. Weeping may be produced by joy, pain, anger, or rage.[37]

What Müller described, then, was how emotion could excite involuntary movement elsewhere in the body. Andrew Hodgkiss has suggested that Müller also envisaged reflexive action as a potentially psychological activity.[38] The German physiologist did indeed allow for the mind to be excited by external stimuli. This was how he perceived ideas to arise, stating that 'an idea or conception is that which is excited in the mind by impressions on the senses, or by those actions of our own body which are communicated to the sensorium'.[39] According to this model, ideas could react upon stimuli originating from outside the body, or from other parts of it. This model was taken up and developed by Thomas Laycock in Britain and Wilhelm Griesinger in Germany, who would suggest that ideas and emotions were not only triggered by external stimuli, but also by activity elsewhere in the body. As will be seen in Chapter 4, Griesinger abstracted from this model an analogous process whereby ideas and emotions would react upon one another, producing novel mental states.

If the brain was subjected to repeated external and/or internal 'irritation', the process of intra-cerebral reflex action would result in persistent mental pain—the manifestation of pathological mood.

THE PHYSIOLOGY OF DISORDERED EMOTION IN MID-CENTURY BRITISH MEDICINE

Kurt Danziger has referred to British physician Thomas Laycock as 'one of the most original minds' among his contemporaries.[40] Laycock left his home county of North Yorkshire to begin his medical studies at University College London in 1833, where he became acquainted with William Benjamin Carpenter when they both attended Robert Grant's optional classes in comparative anatomy.[41] Tom Quick suggests that Grant's lectures helped shape the future research interests of both students, and quotes Laycock as later remarking that 'Carpenter "set on the same researches with himself when both were studying comparative anatomy and physiology".'[42] Having graduated as a Member of the Royal College of Surgeons in 1835, Laycock obtained a position at the York County Hospital the following year. During his time on the female wards at York he published a series of papers on hysteria, out of which emerged his first monograph. *A Treatise on the Nervous Diseases of Women*[43] appeared in 1840, shortly after Laycock received a doctorate in medicine from the University of Göttingen. He was later appointed to the chair in medicine at Edinburgh University, where he would also go on to lecture on metal diseases, remaining there until his death in 1876.[44]

In the 1870s, Laycock and Carpenter would become engaged in a dispute over who had first articulated the idea of psychological involuntary reflexion, or 'unconscious cerebration' as some mid-century British writers called it. The invention of the term 'unconscious cerebration' has been attributed to Carpenter,[45] and he appears to have used it first in the 1842 edition of his *Principles of Human Physiology*. Laycock claimed to have suggested the idea of unconscious cerebral reflexion before Carpenter, first in *On the Nervous Diseases of Women* in 1840, and in a separate article a few years later.[46] The sometimes antagonistic relationship between the two physicians has been engagingly portrayed elsewhere[47]; its bearing upon the present story centres on what unconscious cerebration or involuntary psychological reflexion was meant to convey, how this concept related to Carpenter's term 'ideo-motor' reaction, and what the significance of these models was for mid-Victorian theories of disordered mood.

WILLIAM BENJAMIN CARPENTER

Carpenter developed an impressively substantial framework for physiological psychology in the multiple editions of his widely read *Principles of Human Physiology*, first published in 1842. His theory of mind embraced certain metaphysical principles that set it apart from those offered by Laycock and Griesinger. Carpenter developed a hierarchical table of the nervous system, which also included a division of mental functions. At the lowest level he situated 'the true spinal cord', followed by the medulla oblongata. The next level up was 'the ganglia of the nerves of special sensation', and finally 'the cerebral hemispheres', the latter being the seat of the will.[48] He perceived reflexive action to occur not only in the medulla, but also in 'the ganglia of the nerves of special sensation'. Importantly, involuntary reaction occurring in this higher sphere could be distinguished from the former as it would be 'attended with consciousness, and also, it would appear, with certain peculiar feelings'.[49] This, then, was the seat of emotion (together with the five senses), which for Carpenter had distinctly somatic and animalistic qualities not dissimilar from more traditional conceptions of animal passions and appetites. Volition and emotion belonged to separate spheres in Carpenter's model, and only the latter was prone to the kind of automatism that facilitated physiological theories of insanity. As will be seen below, this was a significant factor setting his framework apart from that developed by Laycock.

According to Carpenter, reactions occurring in the second highest part of the nervous system were 'commonly termed instinctive in the lower animals, and consensual and emotional in ourselves; these all correspond, in being performed without any idea of a purpose, and without any direction of the will, – being frequently in opposition to it'. The result was that in Carpenter's model emotion was a reflexive activity that could occur in conflict with the will. In other words, emotion was something the control of which was at once difficult and desirable, but most importantly *possible*. For volition belonged to a separate, higher sphere, that of the cerebral ganglia, and as such was 'capable of acting in greater or lesser degree, on all the muscles forming part of the system of Animal life'.[50] That is, while Carpenter allowed for psychological reflex action, he perceived it as applicable to 'emotions' and 'instincts', and in later editions of his book to some extent also to 'ideas', but when it came to the will he would not concede to its reduction to a physiological process. In a turn of phrase that brings Hall's dualism to mind, Carpenter suggested that while psychology shared on the whole the same principles as physiology, it was wrong to conceive of 'the Thinking Man' as a 'puppet that moves according as its strings are pulled'. Rather,

> he also possesses a *self-determining power*, which can rise above all the promptings of external suggestion, and can, to a certain extent, mould external circumstances to its own requirements, instead of being completely subjugated by them. We can scarcely desire a better proof that our posses-sion of this power is a reality and not a self-delusion, than that which is afforded by the comparison of the normal condition of the mind, with that in which the directing power of the Will is in abeyance.[51]

It follows from this that a healthy mind would be able to exercise voli-tion to control the other faculties, but in conditions of abnormality, i.e. mental disease, the ability of the individual to direct their will could be compromised. That is, Carpenter insisted on keeping the will sepa-rate from and superior to emotion, but he nevertheless allowed for the possibility of the former becoming compromised by the latter. Carpenter abandoned his tabular division of the nervous system in later editions of his textbook; however, he maintained the separation of the will from the emotions, concluding that, '[t]hat the Emotional and Volitional move-ments differ as to their primal sources, is obvious'.[52] He thus stayed committed to a clear separation of the will from emotion throughout his career.[53] In this way, Carpenter's theory of mind set itself apart from the more strictly biomedical approach of Laycock, as well as that of a new generation of asylum physicians, such as Henry Maudsley, who would apply physiological language to theories of mental disease.[54]

In the 1855 edition of *Principles*, Carpenter attempted to explain the relationship between mind and body through 'a correlation of forces'. There could be no analogy drawn between 'mind' and 'matter'; such a theory was ultimately flawed. However, with the nervous system oper-ating through nervous force, the will could be conceived of as a mental force. In this way, 'nerve-force' could be excited by 'mental agency' and vice versa. This 'correlation of forces' could, he argued, explain the rela-tionship between 'emotional excitement and bodily change', as well as the emergence of ideas in the mind and the subsequent 'action of those ideas upon the centres of movement'.[55] Carpenter assigned this latter operation to the brain itself, giving it the term 'ideo-motor' action. This kind of action was, importantly, both conscious and involving the will in its execution. In this way, Carpenter's model was qualitatively different from the theory of cerebral reflexion developed by his former university associate Thomas Laycock.

THOMAS LAYCOCK

In seeking to explain the 'convulsions', 'fits', and 'paroxysms' of his female patients at York, Laycock drew upon recent research into the physiology of animal bodies with which he had become acquainted during his studies.[56] In *On the Nervous Diseases of Women* (1840), he suggested that most cases of hysteria had an emotional basis, and that the female reproductive system played a central role in producing hysterical fits. Internal, organic actions could, Laycock suggested, trigger a reaction in the brain. Women were particularly prone to such excitability, since their reproductive organs were disposed to causing internal tension and imbalance, upsetting an already weaker and more susceptible constitution. In other words, women were more likely to experience involuntary emotional reactions triggered by external or internal stimuli. Thus, the women's wards at York offered Laycock an optimal stage upon which to observe reflexive emotionality in action. Jacyna observes that '[h]e saw an analogy between [epilepsy] and the "emotional" convulsions of hysteria. It was to explain this analogy that Laycock argued for an extension of the reflex model of nervous action from the spine to the encephalon'.[57]

In *On the Nervous Diseases of Women*, Laycock offered the following description of reflex action:

We find that changes excited in the system by the action of external forces are communicated to the brain by the sensitive nerves; that will act upon the muscles so as to excite motion trough the motor nerves, and that a third class of nerves, the organic,[58] are subservient to the perfection, preservation, and repair of the vital mechanism, and are influenced by certain mental agencies of which we are conscious, – as the emotions, – but which are independent of the will.[59]

Through the class of 'organic' nerves, then, Laycock was able to suggest that cyclical and reproductive changes playing out within the female body could excite the brain and trigger reactions in the form of a range of hysterical-emotional convulsions. However, as we can see, the emotions were correspondingly able to influence bodily functions, independent of volitional control. It was relatively easy for Laycock to proceed from this discussion to drawing a tentative analogy between motor and 'sensorial'[60] reflexion:

> The analogy between the voluntary and involuntary systems of motor and sensitive nerves is partly demonstrated by the previous facts; it remains to inquire whether there be anything in the changes produced in the sensorial system by external and internal stimuli analogous to those excited in the motor. Of these changes it is certain we can only judge by the phenomena produced in each case, *sensation being analogous to movements, abolition of consciousness to motor paralysis.*[61]

This kind of analogy would become central to physiological theories of mental disease. The biomedical language on emotion was riddled with metaphors and analogous explanatory models; as will be seen in subsequent chapters, this language would underpin symptoms of melancholia, such as the ubiquitous 'mental pain' (or *psychalgia*—a term sometimes used to emphasise its analogous relationship to neuralgia[62]). While Laycock displayed some caution in comparing motor and mental reactions, he had little doubt that the brain as an organ was involved in reflexive action, as the 'nervous connexions' running to and from the periphery in his view clearly extended to the cerebral hemispheres. Moreover, he was not blind to the potentially revolutionary implications of such a theory. 'How vast', he exclaimed, 'is the field of inquiry opened out by an application of the laws of reflex function to these structures!'[63] And vast it was indeed. The idea of emotion and even ideas as potentially reflexive, automated, and subject to disorder, has proved one of the most durable legacies of nineteenth-century psychological medicine.

Laycock continued to develop his 'field of inquiry' in his 1844 paper 'On the Reflex Function of the Brain', cited at the start of this chapter. The aim of the paper, he stated, was to 'prove' his earlier claims about cerebral reflexion. Using the example of 'hydrophobia' (fear of water),

Laycock outlined three ways in which such phobia could be induced—
'three classes of irritations [of the brain] inducing the reflex acts of
gasping and spasm of the respiratory muscles'. The first two involved
either the sight of water or bodily contact with it. The third referred
to 'an idea excited by the sound of water dropping, or by the mention
of water'.[64] Once the fear of water—an emotional reaction—had been
induced, the patient 'immediately attempts to remove it. This movement
is strictly involuntary, and not the result of sensation'.[65] What the reader
was presented with, then, was a process whereby a morbid emotional
reaction producing involuntary muscular movement could be triggered
by an idea alone, rather than by sensory stimuli to the body. Laycock
did not name this process, but it is similar to what Carpenter termed
'ideo-motor' activity, to distinguish it from sensory-motor action. What
Laycock did was to describe the means by which this kind of ideation-
ally induced morbid reaction could occur, again by using the analogy of
involuntary or automatic sensory-motor action:

> [S]ince an infinity of muscular acts are already inscribed within the struc-
> ture of the anterior gray matter of the spinal ganglia, and require only the
> appropriate sensory impression to rouse them into action, so ideas may be
> inscribed and require only sensory impressions to rouse *them*.[66]

Danziger notes that Laycock was able to use these principles to explain
'hitherto puzzling phenomena such as somnambulism, hysteria, impul-
sive insanity, and bizarre religious behaviour.'[67] Laycock described, for
instance, a case of a young girl who began to develop rhythmical spas-
modic muscular movements, which over several days developed into 'a
graceful dance' conducted to the melody of the song 'Protestant Boys',
which the patient claimed to be constantly 'dwelling upon her mind'.
When the music became more 'pressing', this 'impelled her to commence
the involuntary actions'. Laycock explained this phenomenon as caused
by 'centric changes, which had induced this alteration of sensory function, and which had reproduced in fact the idea of the air with such force
that it impinged upon the motor track, and there excited consentaneous
reflex acts, in spite of the utmost volitional effort of the individual'.[68]
As will be seen in Chapter 4, the notion of ideas being inscribed onto
the brain, to be aroused anew at any moment by application of appropriate stimuli, was developed in more detail by Griesinger, who offered

the idiom 'mental storages' for the space where ideas were collected in the brain.

While Laycock and Carpenter were no doubt two of the most influential writers of their generation, similar theories were offered by other British medical scientists in the 1840s and 50s. For instance, William Senhouse, physician and anatomy teacher at St. Bartholomew's in London, offered a model of nervous function adopting a stricter level of materialism than Carpenter while still being less radical than Laycock. Senhouse followed Carpenter in separating the 'sensory ganglia' from the 'cerebral hemispheres', with the former being subject to involuntary reaction. The brain itself Senhouse described as the seat of attention, volition, perception, memory, imagination, and judgement, faculties which were all independent of the lower animal functions.[69] However, the operation of these cerebral faculties could still potentially be compromised, resulting in morbidity:

> In health, the mind combines the impressions received by the two hemispheres, and produces from them single ideas, like as in healthy vision the impressions on the two retinæ give rise to a single perception. In certain forms of disease, however, in which, perhaps, one or both hemispheres are disordered, the same object may produce two separate sensations, and suggest simultaneously different ideas; or, at the same time, two trains of thought may be carried on, by the one mind acting, or being acted upon differently in the two hemispheres.[70]

As will be seen in Chapter 4, this ability of the brain to produce unwanted ideas was a key element in German psychiatrist Wilhelm Griesinger's model of psychological reflex action. Unlike Senhouse, who paid scant attention to emotion, for Griesinger the emergence of morbid ideas was closely related to morbid emotionality and the development of melancholia.

Morbid Sensibility and Morbid Introspection

In the second half of the nineteenth century, models of involuntary psychological reaction and the metaphorical language used to create such models would facilitate a reconceptualisation of melancholia into a modern biomedical disease of disordered emotion. More broadly, psychological reflexion and physiological psychology offered Victorian asylum

2 THE SCIENTIFIC FOUNDATION OF DISORDERED MOOD 53

physicians a range of useful tools with which to explain the maladies of their patients. In *On the Nature and Proximate Cause of Insan*ity (1853) James Davey drew upon Billing's model of mental physiology to suggest that in people suffering from mental disease, the 'nervous power' was easily 'converted into *"irritation"* or *"morbid sensibility"*, and this fact is well illustrated by the origin and progress of almost any case of mental derangement'.[71] This argument was further developed in a series of 'Lectures on Insanity' published in the *Association Medical Journal* in 1855, where Billing's concepts 'morbid sensibility' and 'irritation' were presented as central to the emergence of mental disease, and theories within a metaphorical image of muscle contraction:

> Long continued mental exertion, protracted anxiety, or excessive action of any one or more of the cerebral faculties, lead, ere long, to a morbid sensibility of a portion or portions of the cineritious neurine[72]; this, the source of power, intellectual and emotional, if overtasked, loses, like any ordinary muscle, the capacity to respond duly to the too frequent and long continued calls made on it; and it assumes, therefore, a condition of irritation (excitement without power) which, if allowed to proceed unchecked, or if not relieved, realises all the external indications of mental derangement.[73]

The idea of morbid sensitivity of the brain and the mind equally found an abstract application as a means of explaining an old philosophical idea about the causal relationship between solitary introspection and a melancholy state of mind (potentially leading to melancholy madness). Michael Clark has suggested that Victorian medical psychologists held up 'morbid introspection' as an important factor in the aetiology of mental disease.[74] In Clark's narrative of Victorian psychological medicine, morbid introspection was the factor often seen to distinguish an 'unsound Mind' from 'mental soundness'. Defined as 'the habitual turning of the mind inwards upon itself to the virtual exclusion of external impressions, accompanied by the temporary or partial suspension of will or judgment',[75] physicians agreed that morbid introspection fed an unhealthy imagination, leading certain ideas to become dominant and thus destructive to mental health. In this way, emotionality and obsessive ideas would take over at the expense of volition and rational thinking.[76] Clark's narrative is premised upon a view of insanity where 'the condition of "sound Mind", in which reason and will governed the succession of thought and feeling, was familiarly contrasted with that of "unsound Mind", in which reason and will were at least temporarily in abeyance, and emotion, nourished by imagination, held unchecked sway'.[77] However, within the physiological framework for mental activity embraced by mid-to-late nineteenth-century physicians, such a division could not be so easily made. Emotion and volition were not necessarily seen as separate. This was particularly evident in melancholia, and will be considered further in subsequent chapters. A number of physicians would describe melancholics, especially in the early or non-delusional stages of the disease, as being fully capable of reasoning about their morbid emotionality yet unable to think themselves out of their despair. Indeed, this tension was, so the argument went, what drove many melancholics to commit suicide, as this appeared the only 'logical' solution to their suffering.[78] The adoption of physiological language by physicians writing on mental disease led, if anything, to an increasingly complex view of the human mind, one in which the boundary between normal and pathological was perpetually fluid and contested.

By the 1850s, physiological theories of affective insanity were gaining ground among British alienists. Such explanatory models would become increasingly useful later in the century as a biological, evolutionary view of human nature, and of health and illness, gained wide acceptance within the medico-scientific world, and increasingly also outside it. The internal disease model offered by physiological psychology meant that melancholia could be plausibly explained as a biomedical condition in the apparent absence of structural changes to brain tissue. In other words, within a biological system of knowledge, the lack of visible evidence in the form of lesions did not have to preclude the presence of mental disease. As one British physician put it, 'insanity really is a disease of the brain', and an adherence to a physiological view of the mind must lead physicians to recognise that

> the absence of post mortem evidence, even when it is satisfactorily proved to exist, is no argument against the correctness of this opinion, because such a result may merely arise from the real changes being too minute to be detected by the processes in ordinary use for anatomical investigation.'[79]

Thus, the stage was set for a new generation of medical psychologists who were increasingly concerned with diagnosis and classification of mental disease and who sought to anchor their nascent discipline firmly in the conceptual realm of medical science.

CONCLUSION

This chapter has shown how concepts borrowed from experimental physiology and internal medicine were used to speak about the psychology of emotions in biological language. Terms like 'irritation' used to describe the state and function of organs were applied to the mind within a framework where mental activity was conceptualised as the unseen but presumed activity of the brain. Laycock explained mental operations through the concept of cerebral reflexion and perceived the emotions, together with ideas and the will, as produced in the brain—such reflexive action was, in other words, both psychological and cerebral. Carpenter, however, maintained that the emotions were separate from a higher intellect, which retained some measure of control of the former. This tension between emotion and volition would continue to inform discussions about disordered emotion, and melancholia, and were at the heart of ideas about mental pathology embraced by late-Victorian asylum physicians, many of whom drew on Laycock and Carpenter, as well as on the work of influential psychiatrist Wilhelm Griesinger, whose theories of psychological reflex action and the aetiology of melancholia are discussed in Chapter 4.

Physiological psychology came to inform medico-scientific conceptions of the mind and its disorders in the Victorian period, allowing for melancholia to gradually become reconstituted as 'disordered emotion' and as such a modern biomedical mental disease. The consequences of this event were significant for how insanity was perceived in nineteenth-century medicine, not least as it increasingly blurred and shifted the boundary between healthy and pathological emotions. As will be seen in Chapter 5, towards the end of the century physicians were increasingly concerned with 'simple' or non-delusional melancholia. This did not merely manifest in an expansion of the sphere of emotional disorders, but also, and perhaps in a sense conversely, it facilitated the argument that emotional states which physicians themselves considered to be non-pathological could nonetheless legitimately fall within the purview of psychological medicine. Moreover, the development of a physiological model for mental disease did not only have consequences for conceptions of insanity in the nineteenth century. The model of disordered mood that emerged mid-century has proved durable in modern psychiatry, psychology, and neuroscience. It continues to guide present research into the emotions and their disorders, but more than this, it importantly governs what we perceive emotion to be, both as a central aspect of the human condition, and as a private and intimate experience.

NOTES

1. J. Hawkes, "The Materialism of Insanity," *Journal of Psychological Medicine and Mental Pathology* 8 (1855): 313.
2. Thomas Laycock, "On the Reflex Function of the Brain," *British and Foreign Medical Review* 19 (1845): 303.
3. See e.g. David Cahan, ed., *From Natural Philosophy to the Sciences: Writing the History of Nineteenth-Century Science* (Chicago: University of Chicago Press, 2003); Peter J. Bowler, *Evolution: The History of an Idea* (Berkeley: University of California Press, 1989); Timothy Lenoir, *Instituting Science: The Cultural Production of Scientific Disciplines* (Stanford: Stanford University Press, 1997); Lorraine Daston and Peter Galison, *Objectivity* (New York, Zone Books, 2007).
4. Roger Smith, *Inhibition: History and Meaning in the Sciences of Mind and Brain* (London: Free Association Books, 1992), 15.
5. Smith, *Inhibition*, 15. See also Frank Turner, "The Victorian Conflict between Science and Religion," *Isis* 69 (1978): 356–376.
6. Thomas Dixon, *From Passions to Emotions: The Creation of a Secular Psychological Category* (Cambridge: Cambridge University Press, 2003), 180–203.
7. Fay Bound Alberti has traced the shift from ideas about the heart as the seat of the passions and the soul to the modern perception of the brain as the organ of the mind. As Alberti suggests, despite the pervasiveness of neurological discourses on human emotionality in the modern period, the heart remains as a remarkably durable cultural symbol for feeling, particularly love and affection. Fay Bound Alberti, *Matters of the Heart: History, Medicine, and Emotion* (Oxford: Oxford University Press, 2010).
8. Dixon, *From Passions to Emotions*; Roger Smith, "The History of Psychological Categories," *Studies in History and Philosophy of Biological and Biomedical Sciences* 36 (2004): 55–95.
9. Smith, *Inhibition*, 11–16.
10. Historical literature on degeneration abounds. See e.g. Daniel Pick, *Faces of Degeneration: A European Disorder, c. 1848–1918* (Cambridge: Cambridge University Press, 1989).
11. Ruth Leys, *From Sympathy to Reflex: Marshall Hall and His Opponents* (New York: Garland Pub., 1990), 1.
12. Smith, *Inhibition*, 42–55; Jacyna, "Somatic Theories of Mind," 235–240. David Healy also notes the importance of neurophysiology and the reflex concept for the development of modern psychopathology. David

Healy, *The Antidepressant Era* (Cambridge, MA: Harvard University Press, 1997), 31.

13. Roger Cooter, "The Power of the Body," in *Natural Order: Historical Studies of Scientific Culture*, eds. Barry Barnes and Steven Shapin (London: Sage Publications, 1979), 75.

14. Canguilhem suggests, however, that to make Descartes the founder of the modern reflex concept is to distort what is understood by reflexive action, since 'the concept of reflex consists of more than just a rudimentary mechanical explanation of muscular movement. It also contains the idea that some kind of stimulus stemming from the periphery of the organism is transmitted to the centre and then reflected back to the periphery. What distinguishes reflex motion is the fact that it does not proceed directly from a centre or central repository of immaterial power of any kind. Therein lies, within the genus "movement", the specific difference between involuntary and voluntary.' George Canguilhem, "The Concept of Reflex," in *The Vital Rationalist: Selected Writings from Georges Canguilhem* (New York: Zone Books, 1994), 182–183.

15. Edwin Clarke and L.S Jacyna, *Nineteenth-Century Origins of Neuroscientific Concepts* (Berkeley: University of California Press, 1987); Leys, *From Sympathy to Reflex*. Clarke and Jacyna trace the modern concept back to physicians Robert Whytt and Jiří Procháska in the eighteenth century, and locate the first tentative ideas about reflexion in Ancient Greece. However, they also suggest that 'Hall's work constituted a landmark in the history of the reflex concept' (p. 105).

16. Leys, *From Sympathy to Reflex*, 5.

17. Leys, *From Sympathy to Reflex*, 17–18.

18. For older theistic perceptions of the separation of faculties into a higher and a lower sphere, see Dixon, *From Passions to Emotions*, esp. pp. 26–61.

19. J. F. Payne, "Billing, Archibald (1791–1881)," in *Oxford Dictionary of National Biography* (Oxford: Oxford University Press, 2011), http://www.oxforddnb.com/view/article/2387 (last accessed 6/2/2019).

20. Archibald Billing, *First Principles of Medicine*, 3rd ed. (London: S. Highley, 1838), preface.

21. Billing, *First Principles*, 17.

22. Clarke and Jacyna, *Neuroscientific Concepts*, 103–104.

23. Billing drew inspiration for this model of voluntary and involuntary nerves from turn-of-the-century French physician Bichât. However, Billing found Bichât's distinction between 'animal' and 'organic' sensibility and contractibility unhelpful, as all nervous function was, he argued, 'organic', but carried along either voluntary or involuntary nerves. Billing, *First Principles*, 17–19.

24. Billing, *First Principles*, 18.

25. Billing, *First Principles*, 20.

26. Billing, *First Principles*, 108.
27. Billing, *First Principles*, 109. Emphasis in original. Billing's idea of morbid sensibility should not be conceived of in a strictly modern biological sense; rather, his work must be read against the backdrop of eighteenth-century ideas about 'nervous sensibility', which in turn carry with them older Newtonian conceptions of the body. Billing's work was, like much early- to mid-nineteenth-century medical theory, illustrative of a shift from natural philosophy to modern science that was gradual, patchy (and often idiosyncratic), and where old and new ideas were fused in a number of different ways. For 'sensibility' in eighteenth-century medical writings, see e.g. Anne C. Vila, *Enlightenment and Pathology: Sensibility in the Literature and Medicine of Eighteenth-Century France* (Baltimore: The Johns Hopkins University Press, 1998); George S. Rousseau, "Nerves, Spirits and Fibres: Towards an Anthropology of Sensibility," in *Perilous Enlightenment: Pre- and Post-Modern Discourses, Vol. I: Anthropological*, ed. George S. Rousseau (Manchester: Manchester University Press, 1991), 122–141.
28. Billing, *First Principles*, 109. Emphasis in original.
29. See Chapters 4 and 5.
30. Samuel Solly, *The Human Brain, Its Configuration, Structure, Development, and Physiology* (London: Longman, 1836). See also Herbert Mayo, *Outlines of Human Physiology* (London: Burgess and Hill, 1833).
31. Johannes Müller, *Elements of Physiology: Vol. II*, trans. William Baly (London: Taylor and Walton, 1840 [1837]).
32. Robert M. Young, *Mind, Brain, and Adaptation in the Nineteenth Century: Cerebral Localization and Its Biological Context from Gall to Ferrier* (New York: Oxford University Press, 1990), 88; Jutta Schickore, *The Microscope and the Eye* (Chicago: University of Chicago Press, 2007), 134.
33. Schickore, *The Microscope and the Eye*. For *Naturphilosophie* at the turn of the century, see Robert J. Richards, *The Romantic Conception of Life: Science and Philosophy in the Age of Goethe* (Chicago: University of Chicago Press, 2002).
34. Schickore, *The Microscope and the Eye*, 135. Emphasis in original.
35. Schickore, *The Microscope and the Eye*, 141.
36. Schickore, *The Microscope and the Eye*, 134. For a discussion of Müller's role in the development of an emergent modern brain science, see Young, *Mind, Brain and Adaptation*, 88–92.
37. Müller, *Elements of Physiology*, 933.
38. Andrew Hodgkiss, *From Lesion to Metaphor: Chronic Pain in British, French and German Medical Writings, 1800–1914* (Amsterdam: Rodopi, 2000), 90–91.
39. Müller, *Elements of Physiology*, 1354.

40. Danziger, "Psycho-Physiology," 122.
41. Frederick E. James, "The Life and Work of Thomas Laycock, 1812–1876" (PhD diss., University College London, 1995), 22–24; Tom Quick, "Techniques of Life: Zoology, Psychology and Technical Subjectivity (c. 1820–1890)" (PhD diss., University of London, 2011), 91.
42. Quoted in Quick, "Techniques of Life," 91.
43. Thomas Laycock, *A Treatise on the Nervous Diseases of Women; Comprising an Inquiry into the Nature, Causes, and Treatment of Spinal and Hysterical Disorders* (London: Longman, 1840).
44. author unknown) "Thomas Laycock: Obituary," *BMJ* September 30 (1876): 448.
45. Daniel Noble, *The Human Mind in Its Relations with the Brain and Nervous System* (London: John Churchill, 1858), 90. The concept was also discussed by French physician Fahet, who attributed it to 'an eminent neurologist': M. Fahet, "On some of the Latent Causes of Insanity," excerpts (translated) from *Leçons Cliniques de Médicine Mentale*, Paris, 1854, *Journal of Psychological Medicine and Mental Pathology* 7 (1854): 163.
46. Thomas Laycock, "Reflex, Automatic and Unconscious Cerebration: A History and a Criticism," *Journal of Mental Science* 21 (1876): 477–498.
47. Quick, "Techniques of Life," 81–128.
48. William Benjamin Carpenter, *Principles of Human Physiology* (London: John Churchill, 1842), 229.
49. Carpenter, *Principles of Human Physiology*, 228.
50. Carpenter, *Principles of Human Physiology*, 228.
51. William Benjamin Carpenter, *Principles of Human Physiology*, 5th ed. (London: John Churchill, 1855), 549.
52. Carpenter, *Principles of Human Physiology*, 5th ed., 584. Cf. Alexander Bain's discussion of the relationship between emotion and volition. Bain was particularly concerned with the ability to control external manifestations of emotions, such as facial expressions and bodily gestures. Such 'voluntary' manifestations of emotion could, he suggested, be restrained or suppressed by volitional control, whereas 'involuntary' manifestations, such as blushing, could not. Alexander Bain, *The Emotions and the Will* (London: John W. Parker and Son, 1859), esp. 14–15 and Chapter 4, "Control of Feelings and Thought".
53. Two decades later, Carpenter still retained a belief in a will independent from and superior to emotional automatism: William Benjamin Carpenter, *Principles of Mental Physiology* (London: Henry S. King, 1874), 26.
54. See Chapter 4.
55. Carpenter, *Principles of Human Physiology*, 5th ed., 553.
56. Laycock made extensive use of comparative anatomy and physiology throughout his first monograph.

57. Jacyna, "Somatic Theories of Mind," 237. 'Epilepsy' was at this time a term broadly applied to fits and convulsions believed to have a physical basis. While a relatively common feature described in asylum patients, epilepsy was generally not in itself a considered a sign or a form of insanity by British physicians. A helpful illustration of mid-century conceptions of epilepsy can be found in John Hitchman, "On Epilepsy," *Provincial Medical and Surgical Journal* (1852): 5–9.
58. By this term, Laycock meant 'nerves of the organs'.
59. Laycock, *Nervous Diseases*, 97–98.
60. From *'sensorium'* or *'sensorium commune'*, a term that can be traced back to eighteenth-century physician Jiří Procháska, who used it to describe the point of connection between sensory and motor activity—where one triggered the other. Laycock's use of the term should, however, be distinguished from Procháska's, as the former used it to describe the nerves of sensation at the core—i.e. the brain—as opposed to the periphery; in short, 'the central...termination of a nerve'. Laycock, *Nervous Diseases*, 98. See also e.g. Müller, *Elements*, 937. For Procháska's use of the term, see Clarke and Jacyna, *Neuroscientific Concepts*, 105–106.
61. Laycock, *Nervous Diseases*, 113–114. Emphasis added.
62. Richard von Krafft-Ebing, *Lehrbuch der Psychiatrie auf klinischer Grundlag: für practische Ärzte und Studirende*, 5 Aufl. (Erlangen: Ferdinand Enke, 1893), 308; Thomas S. Clouston, *Clinical Lectures on Mental Diseases* London: J & A Churchill, 1883): 32; Henry Maudsley, *The Pathology of Mind: A Study of Its Distempers, Deformities, and Disorders*, 4th ed. (London: Macmillan, 1895), 167.
63. Laycock, *Nervous Diseases*, 195.
64. Laycock, "On the Reflex Function of the Brain," 301.
65. Laycock, "On the Reflex Function of the Brain," 302.
66. Laycock, "On the Reflex Function of the Brain," 303. Emphasis in original.
67. Danziger, "Psycho-Physiology," 127.
68. Laycock, "On the Reflex Function of the Brain," 304.
69. William Senhouse, "The Physiology of the Human Brain," *Journal of Psychological Medicine and Mental Pathology* 3 (1850): 381–382. For the history of perceptions of the two hemispheres in modern science, see Anne Harrington, *Medicine, Mind, and the Double Brain: Studies in Nineteenth-Century Thought* (Princeton, NJ: Princeton University Press, 1989).
70. Senhouse, "The Physiology of the Human Brain," 383.
71. James G. Davey, *On the Nature and Proximate Cause of Insanity* (London: John Churchill, 1853), 27–28. Emphasis in original.
72. In the mid-1800s, 'neurine' referred to nervous tissue (*OED*). By 'cineritious neurine' Davey meant the grey matter of the brain.

73. James G. Davey, "Lectures on Insanity: Lecture III," *Association Medical Journal* 3, No. 140 (1855): 831.
74. Michael Clark, "'Morbid Introspection'": Unsoundness of Mind, and British Psychological Medicine, c. 1830–c.1900," in *The Anatomy of Madness: Essays in the History of Psychiatry, Vol. III: The Asylum and Its Psychiatry*, eds. William F. Bynum, Roy Porter, and Michael Shepherd, 71–101 (London: Routledge, 1988).
75. Clark, "Morbid Introspection," 73.
76. Clark, "Morbid Introspection," 73–80.
77. Clark, "Morbid Introspection," 75.
78. See Chapter 5.
79. James F. Duncan, *Popular Errors on the Subject of Insanity Examined and Exposed* (London: John Churchill, 1853), 14–15.

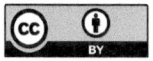

CHAPTER 3

The Classification of Melancholia in Mid-Nineteenth-Century British Medicine

The symptoms of melancholia are so well pronounced when present, and hence so readily recognized, that they do not require to be very minutely described.

J.C. Bucknill and Daniel Hack Tuke (1858)

In 1863 William Sankey, medical superintendent at Hanwell Asylum in Sussex, offered a survey of current perspectives on melancholia in European medicine.[1] One of the first things he noted when comparing works by British, German, and French physicians was the lack of agreement over the nosological status of this disease category:

The foremost question with respect to melancholia is its position in nosology. Some of the authors enumerated[2] ignore its existence as a distinct form of insanity, others retain it as one of the chief divisions of their classification of mental maladies. Now, taking a broad, or what may be called a distant view of the whole, nothing appears more marked or distinct than melancholia from other kinds of insanity.[3]

Sankey's 'distant view' was to become typical of his British cohort in the last decades of the nineteenth century. However, as Sankey's survey indicated, during the first half of the nineteenth century British and European medical literature on melancholia was characterised by divergence rather than coherence. Some physicians, most notably J.C. Prichard, rejected the validity and usefulness of the diagnosis altogether, seeking to replace

© The Author(s) 2021
Å Jansson, *From Melancholia to Depression*,
Mental Health in Historical Perspective,
https://doi.org/10.1007/978-3-030-54802-5_3

it with other diagnostic terms or subsume it under broader categories. At the same time, a reconceptualisation of melancholia began in the early 1840s, a process which would eventually produce a far more standardised and coherent version of this category than had previously existed. This process had its origins in experimental physiology, and emerged out of an ongoing conceptual and terminological shift in the philosophy and science of emotion.

This chapter maps the shifting nosological status of melancholia in mid-century British medical literature, beginning in the 1830s and ending with Sankey's review of contemporary literature on the topic. At the turn of the century, medical writers had begun to argue that the 'passions' played a central role in milder forms of insanity.[4] This idea, emerging before psychiatry itself, proved popular, flexible, and durable. It was foundational to the modern medical concept of disordered mood, and has persisted in some form or another until the present. The twenty-first-century reader must, however, note that to suggest, as Enlightenment physician Phillipe Pinel did, that strong passions can be a cause or symptom of madness, is something quite different from suggesting that emotion is a physiological process prone to disorder and disease.[5] Moreover, it is equally important to note that both these explanations are quite far apart from the twenty-first-century neurochemical model for disorders of mood.

The biomedical melancholia that emerged at mid-century had two important conceptual features, one external and one internal. Externally, it was perceived as a form of mental disease in which emotion was the main, or only, faculty affected, and as such it could present without delusion of thought. An editorial in the *Journal of Psychological Medicine* in 1850 posing the question 'Are delusions always present in melancholia?' is illustrative of this approach. The answer offered by the author[6] was decisive: 'We doubt it. Cases of intense melancholia have come under our notice and care, in which we could not trace the faintest semblance of delusion of any kind'.[7] Internally, melancholia was conceptualised in physiological (functional) rather than anatomical (structural) language as a form of insanity that rarely left visible marks on the brain. In a speech delivered at Hanwell Asylum the same year as the article quoted above, John Hitchman forcefully argued that '*[i]n every case of insanity, there is irritation, or disease of the grey matter in the encephalon*'.[8] He suggested that, while visible lesions may not always be discovered, indeed may not occur at all, mental disease nonetheless always entailed a disorder of brain function. He cited in support of this argument the case of a forty-six-year-old woman diagnosed with melancholia. Her subsequent death was deemed the result of liver failure unrelated to her mental disturbance; the post-mortem examination revealed no abnormalities of brain tissue. This failure to find lesions on her brain was, however, used as a defence of the cerebral theory rather than to rebuke it. The case was presented as evidence of melancholia as a disease of the *physiology* of emotion rather than an illness causing visible and lasting structural damage to the brain.[9]

As discussed in the Introduction, in European medical literature the term melancholia had traditionally been deployed to describe various manifestations of delusional madness characterised by sadness, grief, and despair. Prior to the modern period there was consistently both tension and harmony between medical and lay views of melancholia as madness and melancholy as feeling or temperament. Moreover, in medieval and early modern literature on melancholia and melancholy distinctions were not always made between medical and non-medical descriptions, the most obvious and famous example being the mammoth three-volume ode to melancholy written by sixteenth-century clergyman Robert Burton. While lay and medical perceptions of melancholia and melancholy continued to interact to some extent in the nineteenth century,[10] the two realms grew increasingly separate. This is particularly evident on the pages of asylum casebooks, where patients' expressed religious guilt and fear of divine punishment were generally interpreted and noted down by medical officers as 'religious delusions'. In Victorian Britain, the disease category melancholia came within the purview of psychological medicine (later psychiatry). As such it became a classifiable, diagnosable mental disease with a specific set of symptoms, and often with an expected course of progression. As a disease concept reinvented by physicians wedded to a biological, and specifically physiological, view of health and illness, melancholia was fashioned with a plausible biomedical model that explained in scientific terms how the disease arose. The previous chapter showed how this model was created through an appropriation of language and concepts from experimental physiology, an event that constituted emotion as an automated physiological process. However, the status of melancholia as a distinct mental disease was uncertain in the first half of the century. In part due to the influence of French alienism, particularly the nosological approach of Parisian physician J.E.D. Esquirol, attempts were made to do away with the centuries-old traditional category melancholia. Newer concepts such as 'monomania' and 'moral insanity' threatened to eclipse or even erase melancholia as a diagnostic category in British psychological medicine. However, by the end of the century, melancholia was not only one of the most common forms of mental disease diagnosed in British asylums, it was also one of the most written about in medical literature. Moreover, descriptions of this disease, both in medical texts and asylum casebooks, were remarkably standardised for an age when psychiatry was still in its infancy and no formal standard nosology existed in Britain or elsewhere. This and subsequent chapters constitute an attempt to map how and why this happened.

To tell this story chronologically poses some difficulties, as the reconceptualisation of melancholia was not a linear development. In 1845, influential German psychiatrist Wilhelm Griesinger used his theory of psychological reflexion, which closely resembled Laycock's, to explain the internal aetiology of melancholia in the first edition of his textbook on psychiatry. However, his work was not translated into English until two decades later, and then it was a revised and expanded second edition that finally reached an English readership. At the same time, British writers on mental disease began to appropriate physiological research from the late 1840s, drawing on the works of people like Laycock, Carpenter and Billing. This was, however, a patchy process; biomedical models for melancholia similar to that offered by Griesinger began to gain a foothold in British medical literature in the early 1850s, but many physicians equally continued to favour a more traditional view of mental disease. Griesinger's work and its impact on British theories of mental disease will be considered in detail in Chapter 4. This chapter will begin, however, with the state of British nosology in the first half of the nineteenth century, prior to any significant uptake of physiology into literature on insanity. This is illustrated chiefly by the work of British physician J.C. Prichard, whose major textbook of insanity published in 1835 was largely based on the teachings of Esquirol. The chapter continues into the 1840s and 50s, when British asylum physicians were increasingly embracing models of mental disease based on physiological concepts. Around mid-century, nosological approaches varied, sometimes greatly, yet melancholia was rapidly taking shape as a distinct and easily identifiable disease category, prompting Sankey's conclusion above.

MELANCHOLIA, MONOMANIA AND MORAL INSANITY

When Bristol physician James Cowles Prichard's monograph *A Treatise on Insanity* was first published in 1835 it became part of a relatively sparse catalogue of home-grown British works on mental disorders. While a growing number of public and private lunatic asylums existed around the country in the mid-1830s, standard national guidelines on the management of these were still a decade away. There was as yet no professional association or journal in Britain (unlike on the continent) and universities offered no formal training in what was to become 'psychological medicine' (and later psychiatry). All of this would, however, soon begin to change. Indeed, Prichard himself went on to become one of the first national Lunacy Commissioners in 1845, just a few years before his death. However, at the time when he produced his main work on insanity the landscape of British psychological medicine was still uneven and comparatively barren. Prichard had travelled to Paris and trained under the famous alienist Esquirol, and had become so impressed with the Parisian physician that not only did he attempt to adapt the latter's nosology for a British audience, he even dedicated *A Treatise on Insanity* to his mentor.[11]

Despite a relative scarcity of literature compared to subsequent decades, Prichard's monograph was not the only Anglo-Saxon text on mental disorders available to British physicians in the 1830s. This was a time when the Tuke family's advocacy for moral management of lunatics was gaining ground across the country, perhaps most passionately supported by Prichard's contemporary John Conolly, whose work is considered below. Prichard's classification of insanity, and his approach to melancholia in particular, offers a fitting starting point for the discussion that will unfold in this chapter as it represents a particular early nineteenth-century approach to the classification and diagnosis of mental disease, one which marked itself quite clearly both from traditional medical writings on madness, and the physiologically inspired models that would follow. It was also the by subsequent generations of medical psychologists most read and cited early century British publication on insanity.

While historians have primarily attributed Prichard's place in psychiatry's hall of fame to his supposed invention of the term 'moral insanity',[12] he was also much preoccupied with Esquirol's versatile category 'monomania'. Following Esquirol, he attempted to subsume melancholia under this umbrella category. In doing so, he also classified melancholia as a form of 'partial insanity', a type of madness in which the intellect was only compromised in regards to one particular aspect or idea. This, indeed, was arguably Prichard's more significant contribution to the early creation of diagnostic categories in psychiatry. When the Metropolitan Commissioners in Lunacy (a precursor to the nationwide Lunacy Commission) adopted a formal nosology in the 1840s this included the umbrella category partial insanity under which melancholia was listed alongside monomania and moral insanity. Prichard, however, used partial insanity interchangeably with monomania, and distinguished it from moral insanity. The latter he defined as 'a morbid perversion of the natural feelings, affections, inclinations, temper, habits, moral dispositions, and natural impulses, without any remarkable disorder or defect of the intellect or knowing and reasoning faculties, and particularly without insane delusion or hallucination'.[13] Conversely, monomania (or partial insanity) did involve some measure of intellectual disorder, pertaining to 'one subject, and involving one train of ideas'. The central premise of Prichard's nosological approach was significant: that one could be mad without being fully delusional, an idea that had been gaining ground in medical circles across Western Europe at least since the turn of the nineteenth century.

In addition to Esquirol, Prichard found his inspiration among other European writers, whose work he subjected to critical analysis. He paid a great deal of attention to the early German school of psychiatry, particularly the work of Johann Christian Heinroth, whose view of insanity reflected a Romanticist philosophical worldview. Early nineteenth-century German literature on madness produced in this vein tended to emphasise the importance of the passions (and the soul) in mental disease (Heinroth himself referred to madness as *Seelenstörungen*—disturbances of the soul).[14] However, it was different from the French school in that the latter showed greater interest in the potentially physical basis of insanity; anatomical investigations and particularly psychiatric post-mortems were commonplace in the Parisian hospitals.[15] Prichard attempted to incorporate some of the recent findings of such empirical research, taking stock of the various European writers who had tried to locate madness in brain tissue. His discussion did not, however, move beyond anatomy to take in any aspects of the research emerging at the time in the area of experimental physiology. For the most part, Prichard's approach largely followed that of Esquirol, stating that abnormalities found in the brain tissue of dead asylum patients suggested that insanity was a morbid condition affecting the brain. However, he withheld judgement on whether 'disorders in the affections and feelings' were purely or chiefly cerebral, suggesting that 'however probably it may be thought by some persons that the passions and propensities are seated in the brain, or that modifications which the mind undergoes with respect to these phenomena are connected with instrumental changes in the brain, the fact has never been proved'.[16]

Prichard was primarily concerned with the description of symptoms and the classification of these into correct categories. He suggested of melancholia that it was an outdated term that failed to accurately convey the type of illness it was usually deployed to describe, since 'the illusions which possess the mind are not constantly, in individuals partially insane, indicative of grief and melancholy'.[17] Thus, he concluded that 'Melancholia seemed to be an improper designation for cases of this kind; and the term Monomania, which was happily suggested by M. Esquirol, has been universally adopted in its place'.[18] Prichard was somewhat optimistic in his assessment of the impact of his mentor's nosology; monomania never completely replaced melancholia, but it was taken up by other British writers and became for a while a relatively widely used category in psychological medicine. Esquirol had suggested *lypemanie* ('sadness mania') to denote a melancholic subtype of monomania, but Prichard did not perceive such a specific label to be necessary.

Moral insanity featured at least peripherally as a diagnosis into the second half of the century. Yet, as will be seen in Chapter 5, the nosology favoured by the Lunacy Commission gave primacy to the more well-established categories melancholia, mania, dementia, and general paralysis. Asylum physicians were encouraged to use preprinted forms produced by the Commission to record diagnoses and symptoms, an act that facilitated a gradual standardisation of diagnostics within the significant portion of British psychological medicine that was tied to the asylum. Moreover, the nineteenth-century meaning of 'moral' was ambiguous. While Prichard used the term to mean 'psychological' in the wider sense,[19] conceptualising moral insanity as a form of partial affective mental disease, others used the word specifically to denote insanity that manifested in immoral feelings, thoughts, and actions. James Davey suggested that 'several cases given by Dr. Prichard to illustrate what he conceived to be moral insanity, were instances of everyday mania in which the intellectual faculties had escaped the ravages of the disease affecting the emotional qualities of the mind'. Rather, Davey argued, the diagnosis of moral insanity should be confined to cases where a 'well marked predisposition to the indulgence of the lower feelings and animal desires is manifested'.[20] He deferred to Thomas Mayo's *Elements of Pathology of the Human Mind* (1838) to suggest that moral insanity proper involved an element of 'brutality'.[21] According to Mayo, brutality arose from a 'defect' in 'the emotive department', but he did not consider this a form of insanity in the strict sense, rather it was one of three types of 'deviation from health in which mental phenomena predominate'—the other two being insanity and idiocy.[22] It is important to note, too, that both Mayo and Davey associated brutality and moral perversion—and the emotions more generally—with the lower bodily appetites rather than the higher mental faculties. This is an apt illustration of how older philosophical and medical concepts were fused with the new sciences in this period. The language used to talk about human activity was ambiguous in this sense, with 'emotions' at times being used interchangeably with 'passions', at times to denote bodily 'appetites', and other times as an umbrella term for all mental activity that was considered to have a somatic basis, separate from the intellect.

This oscillation between old and new language was particularly evident in aetiological descriptions. Prichard's account of how a person would become affected by the melancholic subtype of monomania is a case in point:

> An individual of melancholic temperament, who has long been under the influence of circumstances calculated to impair his health and call into play the morbid tendencies of his constitution, sustains some unexpected misfortune, or is subjected to causes of anxiety; he becomes dejected in spirits, desponds, broods over his feelings till all the prospects of life appear to him dark and comfortless.[23]

The idea of a 'melancholic temperament' gradually declined later in the century, but a belief in the predisposition to certain forms of mental disease was maintained by late Victorian physicians through narratives of heredity. In the first half of the century, however, the holistic language of temperament took precedence over a physiological aetiology emphasising cerebral morbid processes in descriptions of melancholia. This was even more prominent in Mayo's discussion of mental disease, where the language used to describe the different forms of insanity was explicitly humoural. Mayo deployed the simple tripartite division of mania, melancholia, and dementia, respectively associated with 'sanguine', 'bilious', and 'leucophlegmatic' temperament. Overall, however, Mayo devoted scant attention to melancholia, including only one case study of the disease in his textbook.[24]

Like Prichard, Davey did not find melancholia particularly useful as an independent disease category, suggesting that '[m]any patients said to be suffering from melancholia labour, in point of fact, under mania; but, in these cases, the most prominent symptom is grief'. In other cases, melancholia was best understood as a form of moral insanity in the broad psychological meaning adopted by Prichard.[25] A point upon which Davey clearly set himself apart from both Prichard and Mayo, however, was in regard to the internal explanation of mental disease, where he adopted a physiological perspective. As noted in Chapter 2, Davey based his theory of disordered emotion and ideation upon Billing's work, suggesting that the latter 'demonstrates that "the consequence of the brain or spinal cord becoming in a state of morbid sensibility is, that their healthy actions are deranged"'. In language similar to that used by Laycock in the previous chapter, whereby abstractly described psychological states could produce morbid physiological reactions in the brain, Davey concluded that '"mental excitement", such as anger, grief, fear, etc., which are analogous to the direct irritation of the brain or spinal cord by a depressed fracture or spicula of bone' would, if carried on over time, result in a 'state of morbid sensibility of the nervous centres'.[26]

'Depression' as a Symptom of Melancholia

Davey's reference to a 'depressed fracture' as an analogy to describe a brain in a state of morbid sensibility manifesting in depressed mood illustrates the multivalence of 'depression' as an emotional state in this period. In the second half of the nineteenth century, depression was increasingly constituted as one of four defining criteria of melancholia (the other three being mental pain, suicidality, and religious delusions, all of which are considered in Chapter 5). While the Oxford English Dictionary dates 'depression' back at least to late fourteenth-century astronomy,[27] the term grew in popularity as a descriptive word in the modern period, and was used throughout the nineteenth century to denote a range of events and conditions. How the term entered the vocabulary of psychological medicine is uncertain; it was at least in part derived from the language of internal medicine, where it was used to speak of the action of the heart.[28] From the turn of the nineteenth century depression gained significant popularity as a term used to talk about a slump in economic markets, and its gloomy connotation in this context cannot be ignored. 'Depression of spirits' was sometimes used to describe a melancholy state of mind prior to the nineteenth century, but as such was conceptually different from the 'mental depression' often referred to in Victorian medico-psychological literature on melancholia.

As noted in the Introduction, the regular use of 'mental depression' to describe the general emotional state of the melancholic in the nineteenth century has led twentieth- and twenty-first-century scholars both in the human and natural sciences to attempt to equate melancholia with the condition commonly known as clinical depression or Major Depressive Disorder in the present. For nineteenth-century physicians, the term was applied in a way that suggested a much more literal meaning, that of something being 'pressed down'. In melancholia, the 'tone' of the mind was slackened and subdued. The mental depression was one in which the operations of the brain were dampened, lowered. This pressing down of the mind was often seen as mirrored in overall bodily function, with digestion, respiration, and movement significantly slower than normal in cases of severe melancholia. Towards the end of the century London physician Charles Mercier suggested that melancholia was characterised by a 'depression of spirits' with a corresponding deceleration of bodily functions:

> We find, therefore, that in melancholia there is evidence of want of vigour in all the bodily processes. The hair grows but slowly, the nails seldom want cutting, the mouth is dry, the digestion is sluggish, the bowels are constipated, the pulse is feeble, the breathing is shallow, the muscles are flabby, the bodily activity is diminished. Together with these bodily manifestations goes a depression of spirits which varies in degree from a trifling want of buoyancy to the profoundest misery and despair.[29]

Victorian medical psychologists spoke of a 'depression of spirits', or an 'emotional' or 'mental' depression when describing melancholia, but the term was predominantly used as a way to describe the overall state of the melancholic mind, and as a way to contrast melancholia with mania—the opposite state of 'mental excitation'. In this way, depression was a helpful concept in the process creating boundaries of classification, but it was not used in place of melancholia, as a term denoting a specific disease.

FROM CONOLLY TO SANKEY: REMAKING MELANCHOLIA

In 1846, British physician John Conolly gave a series of lectures at Hanwell asylum, where he held the position of medical superintendent prior to Sankey. Conolly is perhaps best known to posterity as a vocal champion of non-restraint (and, later, as Henry Maudsley's father-in-law). However, as a well-known and influential asylum physician Conolly was also an important source of knowledge about the diagnostics of mental disease for students and younger practitioners. His 'Clinical Lectures on the Principal Forms of Insanity' were subsequently published in *The Lancet* over several issues. Of the different types of madness addressed, Conolly awarded the most attention to melancholia, the discussion of which constituted three separate articles.

Conolly remained consistent with earlier works in that he did not classify melancholia as an independent disease category, suggesting instead that it was a 'variety of maniacal affection'. Nevertheless, he devoted a significant amount of space to melancholia, and argued that the nature of the symptoms exhibited warranted a separation of melancholia from other types of mania when explaining how to identify and diagnose it. Conolly's descriptive language displayed a mixture of old and new terminology that was characteristic of his generation. On the one hand, he suggested that melancholics were so predisposed because of their 'temperament' and that they could usually be identified according to certain characteristics of 'physical appearance' such as 'dark hair and eyes', 'long features', and 'a sallow complexion'. On the other hand, he incorporated modern medical language when describing the psychological features of the disease, emphasising the key symptom as 'depression of mind'. When discussing the aetiology of melancholia Conolly was chiefly concerned with 'moral' causes, these being 'grief,' 'care', 'distress', 'religious despondency', and 'conscientiousness in excess'.[30] As with the symptomatology of the disease, there was evidence of biomedical language, though it remained unspecific. He suggested that while the illness could be triggered by such moral causes as mentioned above, more often melancholia creates its own distresses, coming on without adequate moral cause, some state of the brain being induced by which it is incapable of receiving pleasing impressions. This state is sometimes obviously connected with morbid actions or conditions of the liver, of the heart, of the intestinal canal, or of the uterus; but oftentimes the cause is wholly obscure; and the unexplained disposition to sadness hereditary.[31]

The framework for this description originates with physiological psychology, where both internal and external sensations could cause an automated emotional response. The idea that morbid action elsewhere in the body, for instance the uterus, could trigger a negative reaction in the brain leading to low mood echoes Laycock's discussion of nervous disorders in women a few years earlier. Conolly did not cite his influences, but he was writing at a time when the ideas of people like Laycock and Carpenter were gaining popularity among British physicians with an interest in mental disease. While not explicitly referring to reflexive action, Conolly drew upon this model to explain instances of melancholia apparently unmotivated by external causes. Going one step further, he also suggested that a mental depression of the mind triggered internally need not be linked to morbidity in a specific organ, but could be due to 'obscure' causes. Conolly did not elaborate further on what such causes might entail; however, his mention of heredity signalled a move towards a concept which would become important to all forms on insanity, as well as to criminality and vice, in the second half of the century.[32] It is also important to note that his argument that the melancholic brain was 'incapable of receiving pleasing impressions' would be modified by later medical writers. As will be seen in subsequent chapters, the increasingly standardised description of melancholia that emerged in the second half of the century generally held that all impressions received by a morbidly sensitive brain, whether positive or negative, would produce feelings of displeasure.

Joseph Williams, a privately practising physician who primarily treated wealthy outpatients, was inspired by Conolly's work and largely followed his approach to the aetiology and classification of melancholia, bringing together traditional language on insanity with modern scientific research. Williams trained briefly at a number of hospitals around Europe and proceeded to bring together his observations and research in an 1852 textbook that situated him somewhere between early century alienists like Prichard and the new generation of medical psychologists who approached their profession and its objects of research from a strongly biomedical viewpoint. His view of mind and emotion was particularly coloured by traditional language. He perceived a division between on the one hand 'emotions', 'passions', 'propensities', and 'bodily appetites', and on the other the 'intellectual faculties' including the will.[33] Contrary to the suggestions of some writers, he argued, 'judgment is always perverted in insanity, although in different degrees.'[34] Moreover, like Conolly Williams perceived a close link between insanity and 'temperament', suggesting that 'those with intensely black hair and eyes are of a nervous temperament and are more subject to melancholia'.[35]

Williams largely adhered to the classification of insanity put forward by the Metropolitan Lunacy Commission in the 1840s. As noted above, this system saw melancholia situated as a subcategory under 'partial insanity', alongside monomania and moral insanity. This nosology was maintained with the creation of the nationwide Lunacy Commission in 1845, and would dominate for a few decades (though monomania and moral insanity were gradually phased out). It is not surprising, then, that a number of physicians writing in the 1850s and 60s adopted this system of classification, regardless of their aetiological approach to mental disease. Moreover, as discussed in Chapter 5, this gradual standardisation of diagnostic categories occurred despite resistance from the Medico-Psychological Association to formally adopting a standard nosology.[36]

One of the early presidents of the Association was Henry Monro (son of the famous Bethlem physician Thomas Monro), a consulting physician on mental disease at St. Luke's whose experience in diagnosing insanity led him to publish several works on the topic. He is of particular importance to the present story as his *Remarks on Insanity* (1851) was one of the earliest British works to fully embrace a view of mental disease firmly anchored in physiological psychology. Monro's adoption of a biomedical model for melancholia and other forms of insanity was rationalised through a now familiar type of analogy. If one believed that mental disease was a disorder of nervous function, one would, he argued, naturally seek to discover 'how far the mental excesses and deficiencies of insanity could be accounted for by the same rules that account for spasm and paralysis of motion'.[37] While the abstract qualities of mind might differ from strictly somatic functions such as 'motion' and 'nutrition', Monro held that that since these distinct functions nonetheless used a common instrument, – namely, nervous matter, and as this mechanism is of the same nature, subject to the same infirmities, and intimately connected in its various parts both by sympathies and continuity, we must believe that, *so far as the various phenomena presented through nervous instrumentality are really dependent on this similar mechanism*, similar results are to be anticipated.[38]

Like Conolly, he also perceived a causal relationship between somatic and mental operations, whereby a disturbance in an organ elsewhere in the body could reflexively trigger a painful cerebral reaction.[39] A healthy mind was one where a 'static condition of the nervous system' was maintained, and where a mental reaction would only occur when 'it is called forth into action by its own proper stimuli'. Conversely, a morbid condition 'is that wherein abnormal stimuli set in action and produce the same effects that proper stimuli should'.[40]

Following from this, Monro put forward a five-point definition of 'the pathology of insanity' based on a psycho-physiological model of mind and brain. He suggested that mental disease constituted 'an affection consequent on depressed vitality', and that 'when the cerebral masses are suffering from this condition of depressed vitality, they lose that static equilibrium of the nervous energies which we call tone'. This muscle metaphor used by Monro to illustrate the state of healthy nervous and mental function became popular with the next generation of medical writers whose work is considered in subsequent chapters, and was deployed to suggest that the 'tone' of the brain was slackened or lost.[41] The analogous relationship between the physical and the mental was then further reinforced by Monro through the suggestion of a reversal of the causal relationship in which 'coincidentally with this want of tone, manifested in the seat of the sensorial faculties, there exists very frequently in the insane a marked want of vitality and nervous tone in those parts of the system which are connected with physical life', such as the skin.[42] In sum, then, somatic disturbances would often give rise to morbid mental reactions leading to or constituting insanity, a condition of lost equilibrium and 'tone' of the cerebral nervous tissue. When the tone of the mind and brain was diminished or lost this would subsequently often lead to an externally manifest loss of tone, such as of the skin or muscles.

When it came to diagnostics, Monro found distinct categories of mental disease less useful than a division of stages into 'acute', 'chronic', and 'imbecile', suggesting that any more detailed and precise distinction was difficult to maintain in a clinical setting.[43] Nevertheless, he proceeded to divide insanity into a number of categories and subcategories. On the status of melancholia as an individual diagnostic category Monro largely followed the recommendations of the Lunacy Commission, including it under the heading 'partial insanity', suggesting that it could manifest without delusion of thought. The description he offered was heavily anchored in the new biomedical language. Melancholia was, he suggested, a condition in which there was a 'general and extreme prostration of all nervous and physical power'; in other words, a 'depression' of nervous power and consequently of mood. In this type of disorder,

the patient does not manifest any delusion until his lowness becomes excessive and more than ordinary, and then his extreme depression runs into terror and anxieties which have no real source; every effort is performed with morbid dread, even the least movement seems sufficient to raise anxious fears; sounds are listened to with anxiety, objects of sight cause an extremely morbid interest: this is a state, in short, of distressing sensibility, which only occasionally runs into real aberration of mind.[44]

Melancholia, then, was chiefly a disorder of affectivity, which in the more advanced stages could also manifest in delusion of thought. Later in the century physicians would generally distinguish more clearly between the non-delusional and delusional forms of the disease by referring to the former as simple melancholia. It would be argued by Henry Maudsley and others that the suffering tended to be greater in this form of the disease, as subjects were fully aware that their mental pain was unfounded and irrational.[45]

A model very similar to Monro's was presented a few years later by George Robinson, asylum physician and lecturer in mental disease at Newcastle. Robinson explained the mind-body relationship by perceiving the brain as the medium between the two, meaning that its health or illness was subject to both mental and physical disturbances.[46] In other words, the brain could be excited by psychological factors—recall the 'mention' of water in Laycock's example of hydrophobia discussed in Chapter 2—as well as by known or unknown activity elsewhere in the body. Robinson was, however, quick to caution his peers against presumption and speculation, warning that 'the precise laws regulating in individual cases the production of the various forms of functional nervous disorder' were 'as yet very imperfectly known.'[47] However, there was, he argued, 'one law explanatory of a large and important group of nervous affections which must not be passed over in silence, namely, the law of reflex action'. From the basic sensation-motion reflex Robinson perceived two analogous laws; the first being

> that the morbid impression produced by a source of irritation existing in a distant part of the body, may be transmitted by the incident nervous fibres to the spinal cord and brain, and thence reflected to various motor nerves, giving rise to convulsions and other results of disordered nervous action.[48]

Following from this, the second law was, he suggested, 'less capable of direct experimental demonstration', but no less central to understanding the emergence of mental disorders. According to this law, 'reflected morbid stimuli' would 'give rise to painful affections in parts far distant from the original seat of irritation, as for instance, in some forms of neuralgia, in sick headache from indigestion, &c'. While having warned against careless conjecture, Robinson nevertheless ventured a third possible law derived from the sensory-motor reflex concept. This was the process ordinarily referred to as 'the association of ideas'. For what was this process, he asked, 'but a species of *reflected feeling*, which from the most trivial circumstances can call into existence, and evolve, an elaborate chain of thoughts and sentiments, apparently the most remote and unconnected?'[49]

Just like sensation, then, emotion could travel as an automated reaction and trigger 'an elaborate chain of thoughts and sentiments'. In a similar fashion to the models offered by Griesinger and Laycock, this analogy described by Robinson largely erased any hierarchical separation between emotion as somatic and ideas and volition as cerebral. Rather, the functions of the mind were, according to Robinson, the result of operations of the brain, which in turn equally depended upon activity elsewhere in the body. A reflexive relationship existed between mind, body, and brain in conjunction, and between emotion and ideas as products of this relationship. It is easy to see how this framework allowed for a range of aetiological explanations for insanity, and specifically for a conceptualisation of disordered emotion as a form of mental disease.

It follows, then, that Robinson believed melancholia to arise from a number of factors, and that this disease did not necessarily entail delusion of thought and judgement: 'Some patients display merely lowness of spirits, with a distaste for the pleasures of life, and a total indifference to its concerns. These have no disorder of the understanding, or defect in the intellectual powers', while others 'derive their grief and despondency from some unreal misfortune which they imagine to have befallen them'. Robinson, too, deployed a nosology similar to the one sanctioned by the Lunacy Commission, which saw melancholia fall under the category 'partial insanity' together with monomania and moral insanity. However, he perceived a much more marked distinction between these three forms of disorder than many other contemporary writers. Taking the literal (and, following Esquirol, original) definition of monomania, he described it as a form of insanity where the patient's intellect was compromised only in relation to one 'particular topic', this frequently being the idea that 'they hold conversations with supernatural beings.' Moral insanity, on the other hand, was often free of delusion, but manifested in 'a total want of self-control, with an inordinate propensity to excesses of various kinds.'[50]

As we have seen, mid-century medical writers were increasingly turning to physiology for language and concepts with which to explain mental disease. This shift was particularly apparent in the work of Daniel Noble, medical officer at a private lunacy facility in Manchester, where he also lectured in mental diseases at the Chatham Street School of Medicine. His *Elements of Psychological Medicine* (1853) acknowledged a significant intellectual debt to Carpenter's work, and appropriated much of the latter's framework for mental physiology. Noble based his theory of mental disease on a psycho-physiological framework of the mind and brain, in which ideas, emotions, and actions could arise reflexively, without external stimuli.[51] However, he departed somewhat from Carpenter's model in designating the different mental faculties to their correct physical location. While Carpenter had assigned emotion to the 'the ganglia of the nerves of special sensation',[52] Noble suggested that it inhabited its own specific space separate from 'the sensibility of the five senses', namely in 'the Optic Thalami and Corpora Striata'.[53] It was evident, Noble argued, from 'the speciality of emotional sensibility' that emotion must originate in 'proper nervous centres'. The reactive power of emotion was significant, he argued, and actions would 'often arrive immediately and exclusively from this inner sensibility'.[54] It is not surprising, then, that Noble was unequivocal in suggesting the possibility of 'emotional disorder' in which there was 'no perversion of ideas'. However, Noble was equally firm in the view that he would 'never characterise such cases as insanity, so long as the reason evinced itself unimpaired.'[55] Where, then, did that leave melancholia? Here, Noble set himself apart from many of his peers in suggesting that cases of 'melancholic depression' of limited duration and where reason was left fully intact should not be considered pathological.[56] Morbid melancholia, he argued, was a state characterised by 'a fixedness and permanence in the moral depression' in which 'the ideas' would 'sustain perversion'. However, in summing up the differences between non-pathological melancholy and melancholia, Noble's description of the latter resonated with contemporaneous views:

> In melancholia, the circumstances are disproportionate to the result; and the ulterior development of the emotional state, becomes referable, very often, to classes of ideas that have no immediate relation with the primary facts occasioning the mental distress; the moral disposition, in other respects, is found to have undergone some notable change, not to be accounted for by ordinary influences; and, moreover, there are often physical signs of nervous irritability or cerebral disturbance.[57]

The view that melancholics tended to attribute an incorrect cause to their suffering would be cited repeatedly by medical writers later in the century. While twenty-first-century scholars have described melancholia in this period as 'sadness without cause',[58] this is a slight misconception of how Victorian physicians perceived it. They distinguished between external and internal causes—the former would usually be (wrongly) suggested by patients, whereas the latter could be correctly assigned by the medical psychologist.

As the works discussed above indicate, during the 1850s the landscape of British psychological medicine was rapidly growing fertile as an increasing number of physicians decided to turn their experience in the diagnosis and observation of mental disease into educational publications. One textbook would, however, tower over other contemporary literature on the topic. Appearing in several editions throughout the early second half of the century, Bucknill and Tuke's *Manual of Psychological Medicine* was one of the most widely circulated textbooks on insanity of the mid-Victorian period, and Tuke's equally impressive *Dictionary*[59] published in the 1890s saw contributions from a range of Britain's most prominent medical psychologists. With the *Manual*, Tuke and Bucknill gave British physicians their most comprehensive textbook on insanity since Prichard's *Treatise*. Indeed, it was the authors' own explicit aim to replace this book with a more modern publication on the topic.[60] They offered a wide-ranging survey of medical opinion on insanity from ancient times until the present, paying particular attention to recent works by home-grown physicians such as Conolly and Monro.

However, remarkably little space was devoted by the authors to the physiology and pathology of mental disease. The reason for this was alluded to by the cautious attitude displayed towards the promise and potential of recent empirical research. Despite what they perceived as great advances in internal medicine more generally, Tuke and Bucknill held fast to the view that the true functions of the brain and their correlation with mental phenomena were in all likelihood perpetually beyond the grasp of human knowledge. Following from this, they were highly critical of physicians who tried to attribute all mental disease to one particular type of disturbance of nervous function, such as 'exhaustion', 'irritation', or 'inflammation'. However, in a broad sense they agreed that all forms of insanity, being disorders of the mind, were also disorders of the brain, and 'that *diseased conditions which affect the mental functions must have their seat in the grey matter of the cerebral convolutions*'.[61] Importantly, the authors did not perceive a division between higher and lower mental faculties, suggesting instead that the brain was the seat of emotion as well as of the intellect.

The model of emotion as a reflexive function of the brain prone to interact with ideas in a similarly involuntary manner formed the basis for Tuke and Bucknill's explanation of the mental suffering typical in melancholia. The despondency of melancholics tended to be at its worst in the early morning, they argued, and this could most likely be attributed to

> the unwonted activity and force which attend all operations of the mind at this period. Every one must have observed the vividness with which suggestions occur to the mind, and ideas irresistibly succeed each other, when conscious, although involuntary cerebration is then first put in action.[62]

Like other authors at the time, they were of the opinion that melancholia could be present with or without delusion of thought and judgement.[63] The authors largely adhered to the nosology endorsed by the Lunacy Commissioners; however, they suggested following Esquirol and Prichard that melancholia could in fact be seen as a type of monomania. However, later editions of Tuke and Bucknill's *Manual* would place stronger emphasis on a biomedical perspective, as well as on melancholia as a distinct disease entity.

Continuing this trend, John Millar's *Hints on Insanity* (1861) reflected several contemporaneous developments, drawing together a physiological explanatory framework with a system of classification that gave prominence to melancholia, mania, and general paralysis. Millar's monograph also contained extensive helpful notes on how to fill out the medical certificates of insanity that were required for the admission of patients under the 1845 Lunacy Law. In regards to melancholia, Millar suggested that there was 'frequently no mental aberration detectable', reaffirming the view that the disease could manifest without delusion.[64] For the most part, Millar's brief monograph consisted of disseminating existing views. However, his discussion of melancholia contained an observation that was at this time relatively peripheral in medico-psychological literature, but which would a mere two decades later be widely accepted as a medical fact, as will be seen in subsequent chapters. 'Every case of melancholia', Millar suggested, 'should be looked upon as having a suicidal tendency.'[65]

As the works discussed in this chapter suggest, when William Sankey published his survey of current medical opinion on melancholia in 1863 something of a coherent approach was beginning to emerge. In published material there was growing agreement on the validity of a biomedical approach to mental health and disease, and the view of emotion as cerebral and subject to disorder was becoming widely accepted. While disagreement on the nosological status of melancholia prevailed, descriptions of the disease were becoming increasingly distinctive as well as comprehensive. When Sankey arrived at his own observations on this disease category, then, the model he offered was firmly anchored in biomedical language. Beginning by discussing the 'excitory-sensatory' and 'excitory-motory' action of the central nervous system, he arrived by analogy at a concept similar to that of Laycock's cerebral reflexion, suggesting that 'illusions' occurred through a mental process analogous to that which produced 'convulsions'.[66] The cause of these 'illusions' (by which is taken to mean the mental or ideational correlate of a physical convulsion—essentially a convulsion of ideas) was 'an abnormal (state) in the nutritive changes of the nervous centres'.[67] The physiological model suggested by Sankey to explain the emergence of disordered emotion was carried over into his description of melancholia as a diagnostic category. He described melancholia as 'a group of morbid phenomena or symptoms......characterised chiefly by depression of spirits'. Sankey went on to list various manifestations of morbid emotion displayed in melancholia, such as mental pain, fear, depression, despondency, selfishness, and suicidal intentions.[68] In this way, Sankey and his contemporaries tried to solve the problem of how to wed a scientific, biomedical model of mental disease with the external manifestations of the patients they encountered by describing an increasing number of the 'symptoms' observed in a language compatible with the internal disease model.

CONCLUSION

Sankey's attempt to reconcile the new biomedical language of disordered emotion with the diagnostic picture of melancholia highlights a conundrum that would pursue medical psychologists throughout the rest of the century. At the same time, however, the language of physiology was making itself increasingly evident in the external symptomatology of melancholia. As this chapter has documented, psycho-physiology gave rise to a new language for descriptive psychopathology, where symptoms such as 'mental pain' and 'depression' were perceived as key features of melancholia. While these symptoms began their life in medical literature, physicians claimed with increasing regularity to observe them in melancholic asylum patients.

The argument that melancholia could present completely without delusion of thought or moral judgement was gradually assuming the status of medical fact at mid-century. Such a belief was in part facilitated by a model of the mind in which the emotions were able to interact and react with ideas. Some writers maintained a hierarchical separation between emotion and intellect, but allowing for the ability of these faculties to interact and react within a framework that nevertheless constituted emotion as chiefly psychological. For an increasing number of medical writers, however, emotion was perceived as cerebral. Moreover, for more strict materialists like Laycock all mental functions, being functions of the brain, were subject to involuntary reflexive action. One of the first medical psychologists and asylum physicians to develop a detailed and comprehensive monograph based on these ideas and devoted solely to the mind and its disorders was Henry Maudsley. His monumental *The Physiology and Pathology of the Mind*, first published in 1867, endeavoured to fully bring together existing physiological knowledge of mental operations and show how the pathology of insanity was not a separate scientific discipline, but merely an extension of physiology. Maudsley's first textbook was a work of medicine, but more than this it offered a comprehensive psychological framework for normal and pathological emotion, a framework which merged the languages of physiology, psychopathology, and evolutionary theory. Maudsley was strongly influenced by both Laycock and Carpenter, but also by the biological and increasingly academic research on mental disease that was coming out of the German states in the 1860s. In Germany, psychiatry became a concept, a trade, and an academic discipline earlier than in Britain, a development spearheaded by an ambitious doctor from Göttingen, Wilhem Griesinger. Griesinger developed a model of psychological reflex action at the same time as Laycock, and applied it to his aetiological work on mental disease. As will be seen in the next chapter, he wrote extensively on melancholia, and influenced a new generation of German psychiatrists whose work was strongly neurological in character.

NOTES

1. William H.O. Sankey, "On Melancholia," *Journal of Mental Science* 9 (1863): 173–196.
2. In the article, Sankey discussed recent works by Tuke and Bucknill, Winslow, Griesinger, Neumann, Wachsmuth, Dagonet, Marcé, Morel, and Calmeil.
3. Sankey, "On Melancholia," 173.
4. Philippe Pinel, *A Treatise on Insanity* (Sheffield: W. Todd, 1806), esp. preface, 16–19, 242.
5. See also Thomas Dixon, "'Emotion': The History of a Keyword in Crisis," *Emotion Review* 4 (2012): 338–344 and *From Passions to Emotions: The Creation of a Secular Psychological Category* (Cambridge: Cambridge University Press, 2003).
6. Forbes Winslow was the founder of the journal in 1848 and its chief editor for the next 16 years. See Michael Shepherd, "Psychiatric Journals and the Evolution of Psychological Medicine," *Psychological Medicine* 22 (1992): 18; Jonathan Andrews, "Winslow, Forbes Benignus (1810–1874)," *Oxford Dictionary of National Biography* (Oxford: Oxford University Press, 2004), http://www.oxforddnb.com/view/article/29752.
7. (editorial) "On British Lunatic Asylums," *Journal of Psychological Medicine and Mental Pathology* 3 (1850): 88.
8. John Hitchman, "The Pathology of Insanity: A Lecture, Delivered May 25th, 1850, in the Middlesex County Asylum, Hanwell," *Journal of Psychological Medicine and Mental Pathology* 3 (1850): 520. Emphasis in original.

9. Hitchman, "The Pathology of Insanity," 510–511.
10. One area in particular where this occurred was that of biographical writing. For an engaging study of the role of melancholia and melancholy in the biographical works of British writers in the modern period, see Jane Darcy, *Melancholy and Literary Biography, 1640–1816* (New York: Palgrave Macmillan, 2013). For melancholia and biography in European writing more generally, see Karin Johannisson, *Melankoliska Rum: Om ångest, leda och sårbarhet i förfluten tid och nutid* (Stockholm: Bonniers, 2009).
11. James Cowles Prichard, *A Treatise on Insanity and Other Disorders Affecting the Mind* (London: Sherwood, Gilbert & Piper, 1835), preface.
12. German E. Berrios, "Classic Text No. 37: J.C. Prichard and the Concept of Moral Insanity," *History of Psychiatry* 10, No. 37 (1999): 111–126; William F. Bynum, "Theory and Practice in British Psychiatry from J.C. Prichard (1786–1848) to Henry Maudsley (1835–1918)," in *History of Psychiatry: Mental Illness and Its Treatments, Proceedings from the 4th International Symposium on the Comparative History of Medicine—East and West*, ed. Teizo Ogawa (Osaka: Saikon, 1982); Hannah F. Augstein, "J.C. Prichard's Concept of Moral Insanity: A Medical Theory of the Corruption of Human Nature," *Medical History* 40, No. 3 (1996): 311–343.
13. Prichard, *A Treatise on Insanity*, 6.
14. Johann Christian Heinroth, *Lehrbuch der Störungen des Seelenlebens oder der Seelenstörungen und ihre Behandlung* (Leipzig: Vogel, 1818). Verwey has divided early German psychiatric writers into two camps—'somaticists' and 'psychicists'. However, the former must be distinguished from a later materialist tradition emerging with Wilhelm Griesinger's work in the 1840s (see Chapter 4). Somaticists such as Jacobi still adhered largely to a view of human nature, mind, and brain steeped in Romanticist *Naturphilosophie* and maintained a belief in an independent abstract soul. See Gerlof Verwey, *Psychiatry in an Anthropological and Biomedical Context: Philosophical Presuppositions and Implications of German Psychiatry, 1820–1870* (Dordrecht: Kluwer, 1985), esp. 27–34.
15. According to one view, Esquirol tried (and failed) to locate 'suicide' in the brains of dead asylum patients. See Ian Marsh, *Suicide: Foucault, History and Truth* (Cambridge: Cambridge University Press, 2010), 117–122.
16. Prichard, *A Treatise on Insanity*, 246.
17. Prichard, *A Treatise on Insanity*, 26–27.
18. Prichard, *A Treatise on Insanity*, 27.
19. Cf. 'moral treatment', which was both 'moral' (in today's meaning of the word) and psychological. With the physician as a stern but affectionate father figure, moral treatment aimed to restore lunatics to their rational selves through a combination of kindness, discipline, and light

employment. See e.g. Samuel Tuke, *Description of the Retreat* (York: W. Alexander, 1813), esp. pp. 131–136.

20. Davey, "Lectures on Insanity," 829.
21. The word brutality as used here should be understood as being closer in meaning to its etymological origins than its twenty-first century usage— i.e. as associated with 'brutes'.
22. Thomas Mayo, *Elements of the Pathology of the Human Mind* (London: John Murray, 1838), 148–149.
23. Prichard, *A Treatise on Insanity*, 28.
24. Mayo, *Pathology of the Human Mind*, 66, 111–113.
25. Davey, "Lectures on Insanity," 828–829.
26. Davey, "Lectures on Insanity," 831.
27. For instance: 'And than is the depressioun of the pol antartik, þat is to seyn, than is the pol antartik by-nethe the Orisonte the same quantite of space.' Geoffrey Chaucer, *A Treatise on the Astrolabe: Addressed to His Son Lowys* (London: N. Trübner & Co., 1872 [1391]). Reference derived from the *OED* entry on 'depression': http://www.oed.com/ (accessed 04/05/2013).
28. See Fay Bound Alberti, *Matters of the Heart: History, Medicine, and Emotion* (Oxford: Oxford University Press, 2010), for the shift from the heart to the brain as the centre of feeling, a shift that nevertheless saw the former's significance maintained as a metaphor.
29. Charles A. Mercier, *Sanity and Insanity* (London: Walter Scott, 1890), 337. See also e.g. Henry Maudsley, *The Pathology of Mind*, 4th ed. (London: Macmillan, 1879 & 1895), 164; John C. Bucknill and Daniel Hack Tuke, *A Manual of Psychological Medicine*, 4th ed. (London: John Churchill, 1879), 220–221; George Savage, *Insanity and Allied Neuroses: Practical and Clinical* (London: Cassell, 1884), 152–154.
30. John Conolly, "Clinical Lectures on the Principal Forms of Insanity, Lecture VII," *The Lancet* (January 3, 1846): 1.
31. Conolly, "Clinical Lectures," 1.
32. See e.g. Henry Maudsley, *Responsibility in Mental Disease* (London: Henry S. King, 1874).
33. Joseph Williams, *Insanity: Its Causes, Prevention, and Cure*, 2nd ed. (London: John Churchill, 1852), 4–5.
34. Williams, *Insanity*, 7.
35. Williams, *Insanity*, 39.
36. The Medico-Psychological Association, which originated in 1841 as the Association of Medical Officers of Asylums and Hospitals for the Insane, was the main forum for discussion of clinical, administrative, and theoretical questions for British physicians working in the field of mental disease. See Chapter 5.

37. Henry Monro, *Remarks on Insanity: Its Nature and Treatment* (London: John Churchill, 1851), vii.
38. Monro, *Remarks on Insanity*, vii. Emphasis in original.
39. Monro, *Remarks on Insanity*, 5.
40. Monro, *Remarks on Insanity*, 10.
41. Monro, *Remarks on Insanity*, 12.
42. Monro, *Remarks on Insanity*, 14.
43. Monro, *Remarks on Insanity*, 2.
44. Monro, *Remarks on Insanity*, 27.
45. See Chapter 5.
46. George Robinson, *On the Prevention and Treatment of Mental Disorders* (London: Longman, 1859), 20–23; 43.
47. Robinson, *Prevention and Treatment*, 44–45.
48. Robinson, *Prevention and Treatment*, 44.
49. Robinson, *Prevention and Treatment*, 44–45. Emphasis in original.
50. Robinson, *Prevention and Treatment*, 53–54.
51. Noble adopted Carpenter's concept of ideo-motor action, but suggested that such activity could perhaps be more aptly termed 'ideo-dynamic'. Daniel Noble, *Elements of Psychological Medicine: An Introduction to the Practical Study of Insanity* (London: John Churchill, 1853), 69–71.
52. See Chapter 1.
53. Noble, *Psychological Medicine*, 72–74. Here, Noble departed from a view endorsed by a number of mid-century scientists, who perceived these two regions as constituting the centres of movement and sensation. Robert M. Young, *Mind, Brain and Adaptation in the Nineteenth Century: Cerebral Localization and Its Biological Context from Gall to Ferrier* (New York: Oxford University Press, 1990), 111–113. In the last quarter of the century, experimental physiologists would more firmly suggest their central role in bodily movement. Galvanic experiments on dogs indicated that after removal of the hemispheres, motor action was still possible following direct stimulation if the optic thalami and corporal striata were left intact. See e.g. David Ferrier, *The Functions of the Brain* (New York: G.P. Putnam & Sons, 1876), 214.
54. Noble, *Psychological Medicine*, 76.
55. Noble, *Psychological Medicine*, 180–181.
56. Cf. Maudsley on simple melancholia, Chapter 5.
57. Noble, *Psychological Medicine*, 215–216.
58. Allan V. Horwitz and Jerome C. Wakefield, *The Loss of Sadness: How Psychiatry Transformed Normal Sorrow into Depressive Disorder* (Oxford: Oxford University Press, 2007), 66–71.
59. Daniel Hack Tuke, ed., *A Dictionary of Psychological Medicine* (London: J.A. Churchill, 1892).

60. John Charles Bucknill and Daniel Hack Tuke, *A Manual of Psychological Medicine* (London: J.A. Churchill, 1858), preface.
61. Bucknill and Tuke, *A Manual of Psychological Medicine*, 389. Emphasis in original.
62. Bucknill and Tuke, *A Manual of Psychological Medicine*, 157.
63. Bucknill and Tuke, *A Manual of Psychological Medicine*, 157–159.
64. John Millar, *Hints on Insanity* (London: Henry Renshaw, 1861), 22.
65. Millar, *Hints on Insanity*, 23.
66. Sankey, "On Melancholia," 193–194.
67. Sankey, "On Melancholia," 194.
68. Sankey, "On Melancholia," 179.

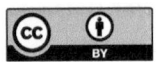

CHAPTER 4

Melancholia and the New Biological Psychiatry

[W]hen there is perversion of the affective life, there will be morbid feeling and morbid action; the patient's whole manner of feeling, the mode of his affection by events, is unnatural, and the springs of his action are disordered; and the intellect is unable to check or control the morbid manifestations, just as, when there is disease of the spinal cord, there may be convulsive movement, of which there is consciousness, but which the will cannot restrain.[1]

Henry Maudsley (1867)

By the 1860s, the concept of disordered emotion as a physiological phenomenon was firmly established in British medicine. The physiological models of mental operations proposed by Carpenter and Laycock outlined in Chapter 2 were foundational for this development. As previously noted, at the same time as Laycock put forward his theory of cerebral reflex action, German physician Wilhelm Griesinger presented an almost identical model which he referred to as 'psychological reflex action' (*psychische Reflexactionen*). While neither Carpenter nor Laycock discussed mental reflex action in relation to depressive emotions, Griesinger applied his theoretical framework to melancholia and disordered mood. His textbook on mental pathology, first published in 1845 with a second, revised and expanded edition reaching a wide European audience in the 1860s, offered one of the century's most influential nosological descriptions of melancholia firmly anchored in a physiological model of emotion.

© The Author(s) 2021
Å Jansson, *From Melancholia to Depression*,
Mental Health in Historical Perspective,
https://doi.org/10.1007/978-3-030-54802-5_4

Griesinger inspired a new generation of physicians in Germany and beyond, including in Britain. In the late 1860s, up and coming asylum physician Henry Maudsley drew on Griesinger's work, as well as on the ideas of some of the most prominent scientific minds of the time, including Laycock and Carpenter, as well as Herbert Spencer and Charles Darwin. Maudsley sought to definitively merge physiology and psychology into a new scientific psychiatry that was equally concerned with classification and aetiology. His model of disordered mood and his nosological system had a far greater impact on subsequent psychiatric knowledge than is generally recognised by historians today. As a new scientific psychiatry was rapidly endorsed across Britain and the continent, numerous voices were added to those of Griesinger and Maudsley. In mapping the development of a biological model for melancholia and disordered mood, this chapter begins by tracing Griesinger's work on psychological reflexion and disordered mood from the 1840s until his premature death in 1868. The chapter then looks more closely at the uptake up these ideas into British psychological medicine in the 1860s, culminating in the publication of the first edition of Maudsley's *The Physiology and Pathology of the Mind* in 1867. Finally, the story travels back to Germany and the model of melancholia presented by Richard von Krafft-Ebing in 1874. The chapter concludes by considering the relationship between melancholia and neurasthenia, in the context of North-American psychiatry in the last quarter of the nineteenth century.

WILHELM GRIESINGER: FROM CEREBRAL IRRITATION TO MENTAL DEPRESSION

As a precocious young student Wilhelm Griesinger travelled around the continent for his medical training, receiving instruction from, among others, François Magendie in Paris.[2] Upon his return to Prussia, he quickly rose among the ranks of a new generation of physicians advocating a scientific, academic psychiatry, and assumed the first combined chair of psychiatry and neurology at Berlin's Charité in 1864. Among his German contemporaries, Griesinger was best known and remembered as the controversial physician who attempted to bring about a radical reform of Prussian psychiatry. His bold modernisation programme presented in 1867 aimed to bring mental disorders out of isolated rural asylums and into a new generation of 'city clinics' situated in close proximity to university hospitals in order to facilitate research and clinical training.

The proposal generated discord within the psychiatric community in the German states, a battle which would continue to rage after his premature death from appendicitis in 1868.[3]

In 1843, a year after completing his psychiatric training under Alfred Zeller at the asylum in Winnenthal, Griesinger published an article entitled 'On psychological reflex action' (*Ueber psychische Reflexactionen*),[4] in which he developed a physiological model of mental reflexion, and discussed its implications for psychopathology. Griesinger constructed much of his physiological model of reflexive action from what had been observed during experiments on living animals and what had been inferred from such research about that which scientists could not see. He suggested that existing experimental data showed that, as well as movements directed by the will, 'one could observe in animals a number of other muscle contractions triggered by centripetal sensory impressions'. Such impressions would, he argued, pass through the brain without alerting consciousness, and would result in muscle contraction being performed 'more completely' than in the case of conscious movement.[5] In other words, unconscious motor reactions were potentially more powerful than those directed by conscious volition.

Griesinger then extrapolated this theory to suggest that involuntary and/or unconscious emotional reactions were more powerful than mental operations directed by the will. Like Laycock, he suggested that ideas could excite motor action as well as emotional reactions and the bodily manifestations accompanying the latter, adding an element that would become crucial to a physiological model for affective insanity. For Griesinger, external stimuli (such as Laycock's 'sound' or 'mention' of water) were not necessary to produce morbid emotion. Ideas kept in mental storages (*geistiges Vorraths*) could spontaneously and internally react upon one another. The 'totality of all exciting factors of [the brain]' was, he suggested, made up of both conscious and unconscious impressions, which were merged together to become new mental representations. That is, the brain stored and fused all impressions received, some of which passed through consciousness, and some which were stored without triggering awareness. All impressions were capable of reacting upon one another, and in doing so could synthesise and create new ideas, or mental representations (*Vorstellungen*), which could emerge endogenously, independent of external stimuli. When new impressions reached the brain from outside, ideas kept in mental storages were able to react upon previously stored images to produce novel ones. In a healthy brain, this process was self-regulating, maintaining the 'tone' of the brain, but in a disordered brain this kind of reactivity was the source of morbid symptoms such as depressed mood.[6]

Griesinger has been hailed as the founder of modern biological psychiatry,[7] but like most of his contemporaries he struggled to make sense of the relationship between mind and brain. In the quest to explain that which verged on the inexplicable, metaphors were an invaluable device for nineteenth-century physicians. 'Tone' was one such metaphor. It was widely useful in nineteenth-century psychological medicine, but has not survived into the present. Tone came for Griesinger to denote both something tangible, like the physical tone of a muscle, as well as a kind of mental harmony, the maintenance of which was a prerequisite for a healthy mind. The tone of the brain, i.e. of the cerebral ganglia, was affected by the nature of mental images (*Vorstellungen*), so that, for instance, 'sad' images could serve to 'slacken' the tone of the brain.[8]

Two things in particular should be noted about Griesinger's physiological explanation of how ideas and emotions were generated in the brain. First, his theoretical framework must be understood against the backdrop of pre-nineteenth-century philosophical models of the mind. As Gerlof Verwey has shown, while Griesinger was explicitly committed to a biological view of mental pathology, there was a strong philosophical undertone throughout his work, which Verwey describes as 'an exemplary manifestation of the link between old and new'.[9] This is demonstrated both by the abstract language used, and more specifically by the description of mental images as reacting upon one another to produce new ones. The latter bears resemblances to eighteenth-century associationist psychology, and would also re-emerge in mid-century Britain, where Herbert Spencer developed similar ideas within a new physiological framework.[10]

Second, the ability of the brain to react both to external and internal stimuli, and to produce from any combination of these entirely new impressions and ideas, formed the basis of a new biomedical model of mental disease. Moreover, as suggested above, for Griesinger it was the *unconscious* ideational reactions that were the most powerful. If an increasing number of negative impressions were stored and subsequently reacting both with further external irritants and with each other internally, the brain would be subjected to repeated 'irritation' [*Reize*]. Eventually, the process of automated or reflexive mental reaction would become disordered. The brain would then begin to produce morbid reactions, such as pathological feelings of displeasure, in response to factors that would not trigger such reactions in a healthy mind.[11] Griesinger's model for describing the internal aetiology of mental disease followed the kind of physiological description offered by Billing and other contemporary European writers such as Müller (see Chapter 2). The 'irritation' of an organ leading it to become more sensitive or, in Billing's words, subject to 'morbid sensibility', served as a plausible metaphor for explaining affective insanity within a biomedical framework. In other words, language used to describe observable disease in organic tissue was now applied to make the unseen and unknown familiar and explicable. The analogous transfer that occurred here was ambiguous. The new physiological language was at once applied to talk about an organ—the brain—and its perceived function—the mind, and the operations of both of these, which, while for materialists like Laycock and Griesinger were perceived as strictly organic, could nevertheless not be observed with the naked eye, but only theorised according to language extrapolated from the observable somatic realm of internal medicine. What occurred here was not, then, simply a transfer from the physical to the psychological, but rather the creation of a new sphere within medical science, one in which physiology and psychology were not merely complementary to each other, but merged into a new system of knowledge.

Griesinger ended his essay by outlining what he perceived to be the implications of psychological reflex action for the study of insanity. In doing so he suggested that there were two basic emotional 'anomalies' which were foundational to all forms of mental disease. One was characterised by an 'elevated sense of self', and the other by a sense of 'dejection' and feeling of 'mental displeasure'. He went on to argue that 'in the infinite majority of cases, almost without exception, the starting point for all subsequent changes in mind which insanity entails are the latter states, those of mental depression'.[12] It follows that he discussed melancholia at length in his textbook on mental pathology. He saw it as the first stage in mental disease, suggesting that it was therefore more treatable than other forms of insanity. The ability of physicians to recognise the onset of melancholia early on was, he argued, essential in order to facilitate early medical intervention. It was therefore imperative that all doctors were able to correctly detect and diagnose this form of insanity.[13]

'PAIN IS AWAKENED BY THE SLIGHTEST
IMPRESSION': GRIESINGER'S MELANCHOLIA

Griesinger favoured a modern version of the traditional tripartite division of insanity into melancholia, mania, and dementia, referring to these as the 'states of mental depression', the 'states of mental exaltation', and the 'states of mental weakness'. He also adhered to the theory of unitary psychosis which held that all forms of madness constituted different stages in the same disease.[14] For Griesinger, comprehensive knowledge of states of mental depression [*Depressionzustände*] was imperative if one was to understand the onset and progression of mental disease more generally. These states, which included hypochondria and simple and delusional melancholia, were discussed at great length in the second extended edition of his textbook on mental pathology.[15]

The view that low mood was the first sign of oncoming mental disease meant that Griesinger argued forcefully for the importance of early detection and diagnosis of this form of insanity, since the progression from melancholia to mania and later dementia and death was a significant risk if symptoms were left untreated. The sooner clinical attention was brought to bear upon people displaying symptoms of melancholia, the greater the chance of rapid recovery.[16] In conjunction with his proposal for urban clinics referred to above, he argued forcefully in favour of clinical training of students and of utilising psychiatric wards as sources of academic research. Psychiatry had to become a medical science, both as a practised speciality and as an academic discipline, and all medical students should receive proper instruction in how to identify and diagnose mental disease so that the milder forms —in other words the first stages of illness—would not go undetected.[17] Central to Griesinger's reform plan was, then, an emphasis on milder forms of insanity—the states of mental depression. It was essential that physicians were familiar with a clear and comprehensive description of melancholia and that they understood what emotional disorders entailed, how they functioned, and how to identify them. Only the physician with proper psychiatric training could be sure to correctly distinguish between melancholia and normal, non-pathological low mood, a view that would often be repeated by British physicians later in the century.

While one historian has suggested that Griesinger 'based his definitions on borrowed cases and views',[18] he drew on cases of melancholia which he had come across when training under Alfred Zeller, as well as cases presented or published by other alienists.[19] More importantly, however, the significance of Griesinger's work did not rest upon the originality of the case studies he produced, but on the biomedical model for insanity he presented. The framework for explaining affective insanity through psycho-physiological reflexion as the basis of disordered emotion would form an invaluable model for explaining affective disorders, particularly melancholia, throughout much of the century. While earlier physicians such as Pinel and Esquirol had begun to talk about 'affective', 'moral', or 'partial' insanity, Griesinger fashioned such disorders with an internal biomedical model which explained *how* emotion could become diseased, using the language of empirical science.

The second expanded edition of *Die Pathologie und Therapie der Psychischen Krankheiten* (1861), which was translated into English, began with a lengthy discussion of brain anatomy and physiology. Griesinger was unequivocal in the view that insanity had organic roots even when visible lesions could not be found, since mental activity was a physiological process, 'a special life form of the organism'.[20] The textbook incorporated sections from his article on psychological reflex action and further elaborated the principles developed in the 1843 paper. In doing so, Griesinger highlighted an aspect of mind that constituted one of the more radical claims to emerge from physiological psychology at this time, and which he was not alone in making. Within a framework where all functions of mind (or, as Griesinger termed it here, '*Vorstellen*,' roughly 'imagination') could be explained through the same physiological principles, the different mental faculties were hierarchically equal.[21] Recalling his model of mental operations discussed above, he held that 'all the various mental acts which were formerly designated separate faculties (fantasies, will, emotions, etc.) are only different relations of the imagination with sensation and movement, or the result of the conflicts of mental representations with themselves'.[22]

This act of constituting emotion, thought, and volition as equal, cerebral physiological processes, formed one of the cornerstones of theories of insanity suggesting that the mind could be diseased without causing delusion, and as such it helped facilitate and make plausible the medical condition 'simple melancholia'. By raising emotion to a level equal with cognition and volition, Griesinger made it possible for automated, unconscious interaction between these faculties to occur. Esquirol's *monomanie* and Prichard's moral insanity had conceptually suggested that in certain

forms of insanity the passions were chiefly affected, and often constituted the cause of mental disease, but these models nonetheless insisted
on some measure of intellectual derangement. The argument that one
could suffer from mental disease without exhibiting any delusion of intellect or compromising of reason constituted a significant shift from earlier
perceptions of what madness was.[23]

Griesinger went on to further develop the analogy of sensory-motor
reaction as a model for how ideas and emotions were produced:

> In the wider sense of the mind….every mental function, active or passive,
> and naturally also emotion, is a form of imagination. Emotion is an imag-
> ination which has arisen in the brain through immediate irritation of a
> centripetal fibre. A great number of mental images are not immediately
> provoked by irritation of the sensitive nerves, but are produced internally
> by the functions of the brain, which are independent of all sensorial exci-
> tation. They are also intimately dependent upon the traces which former
> sensorial impressions have left in the brain, and on the inward phenomena
> of sensation.[24]

As Griesinger had suggested in his article on the mental reflex, this
ability of mental representations to react upon one another internally was
key to understanding how mental disorders emerged. Just as reflexive
action could be triggered solely within the realm of the mind, so was
'irritation' able to occur without external influence. *Vorstellungen* could
be triggered into reaction 'not only by their normal, external irritants,
but also by internal irritation'.[25] Often, internal irritation would have
its source elsewhere in the body, meaning that the immediate cause
of insanity was in many cases some other bodily dysfunction or imbalance escaping conscious awareness. However, even if the original source
of internal irritation was removed, the mental disorder may persist and
develop independently. Moreover, 'such organic irritations do not usually
excite new, clear and definite ideas but, in the first place, they cause those
vague, indeterminate modifications of the mind which we call emotion
(*Gemütsbewegung*)'.[26] The fact that such internal irritation was often not
consciously perceived helped explain, then, why the initial production of
morbid mental action was one affecting emotion before the intellect.

Such morbid cerebral action could then give rise to the kinds of symptoms associated with melancholia. In discussing these, Griesinger again
deployed the analogy of physical sensation, but this time explicitly. Mental

images could, he suggested, be 'accompanied by pain or pleasure'. A disordered mind became subject to 'mental pain', which could at times be specific, linked to a particular mental image, but more often it was vague and diffuse, relating to 'emotion or the intellect as a whole': 'Much like in a bodily state of general pain and discomfort, so in the mind a causeless feeling of trepidation, anxiety, etc., when long continued, will eventually develop painful ideas'.[27] It was in such general mental pain and 'lowness of spirits' which melancholia consisted. Griesinger began his chapter on the 'states of mental depression' by proclaiming that '[t]he fundamental affection in all these forms of disease consists in the morbid influence of a painful depressing negative affect – in a mentally painful state'.[28] Recalling the discussion of 'depression' in Chapter 3, Griesinger was explicit in stating that he did not deploy the term in the strictly medical, physiological sense of lowered function, but as a descriptive term to denote a state of mind. In other words, mental depression did not denote 'passivity or weakness', or a 'suppression' of cerebral phenomena, rather, 'lively irritation of the brain and a commotion of the psychological processes are the foundation of this state; but the collective result of these (cerebral and psychic) processes for the general mood is a depressive or painful state'.[29]

While melancholia was often, as suggested above, initially induced by some form of internal bodily dysfunction subconsciously triggering cerebral irritation, it would at times also appear to be brought about in the first instance by 'normal' sadness or dejection such as 'grief' or 'jealousy'. Griesinger noted the problem of distinguishing the mental pain of melancholia from non-pathological 'painful emotion', but held that it would mark itself as different 'by its excessive degree, by its more than ordinary protraction, by its becoming more and more independent of external influences, and by the other accessory affections which accompany it'.[30] What such 'accessory affections' consisted in depended in part upon which type of melancholia a person was suffering from. Hypochondria, according to Griesinger 'the mildest, most moderate form of insanity', was distinguished by a range of pronounced bodily complaints. These were in addition to 'the generic character of dejection, sadness, depression of mind, diminution of the activity of the will, and of a delirium which corresponds to this mental disposition'. However, in hypochondria 'the emotional depression proceeds from a strong feeling of bodily illness'. While hypochondria resulted in 'false conceptions' the intellect was for the most part uncompromised and the patient was able to follow logical reasoning.

The application of the mental reflex can be noted in the aetiology of hypochondria. The psychological feeling of bodily illness often emerged, Griesinger suggested, through 'irritation of the nervous centres arising from peripheral disease—often very obscured and concealed – of the viscera'. However, the perception of somatic dysfunction would take on a life of its own, persisting and growing independently of any bodily malady, and the more mental attention was focussed on these perceptions of illness, the stronger the feeling of bodily and mental discomfort would become.[31] The states of mental depression would often commence with some measure of hypochondric features, at least if the original trigger for the disease was located elsewhere in the body. If medical attention was not brought upon the person afflicted, this 'state of vague mental and bodily discomfort' would pass into a persistent melancholia proper, characterised by a 'state of mental pain' which would be 'increased by every external mental impression'.[32] This mental pain would soon begin to eclipse every other feeling of the sufferer, consuming every aspect of bodily and mental function. It 'consists in a profound feeling of ill-being, of inability to do anything, of suppression of the physical powers, of depression and sadness, and of total abasement of self-consciousness'. The entire character of the person so afflicted would eventually be transformed. The process by which feelings and ideas were produced would become so distorted, so diseased, that positive thoughts or feelings of joy were no longer possible.[33]

The disease process could equally start not with hypochondria but with simple melancholia. The two were similar in that both lacked the presence of proper delusion; the mind had not been fully consumed by the disease in that patients would be able to reason about their morbid feelings. However, with the physiological process of emotion having become disordered, the will was also affected. While patients were able to understand that their mental pain was unreasonable and unfounded, they were completely unable to master their morbid emotions.[34] They could properly assess the 'objects of the outer world', but these produced 'an impression utterly different from what they were wont to do, of which the intelligent and educated sufferers can alone give a true description. "It appears to me" says such a melancholic, "that everything around me is precisely as it used to be, although there must have been changes."' At first, the patient would be fully aware of this shift in their mental state, '[h]e even complains himself that his sensations are no longer natural, that they are perverted'.[35] Simple melancholia, then, consisted in a state of disordered feeling accompanied by diminished volition. This disease model was made possible by the application of the reflex concept to all mental processes. In this way, the model of psychological reflex action developed by Laycock and Griesinger facilitated a view of insanity in which the idea of pathological emotionality was a plausible medical concept. The idea of disordered emotion as a physiological process was widely appropriated by British physicians in the decades that followed, bringing about a reconfiguration of melancholia in Victorian medicine.

HENRY MAUDSLEY: DISORDERED EMOTION IN AN EVOLUTIONARY CONTEXT

Henry Maudsley published extensively over more than four decades, with the bulk of his publications concerning the mind–body relationship and mental pathology.[36] His preoccupation with mental disorders extended to include insanity and the law, an interest that grew out of his research on the physiology and psychology of 'morbid impulses'. His work was widely read by his peers, both in Britain and on the continent. Maudsley also published more on melancholia than almost any other of his British contemporaries. He embraced a theory of mind heavily anchored in physiological psychology, emphasising the significance of the 'latest advances in physiology, and....the present state of physiological psychology in Germany', drawing a parallel between research emerging from the German states and the theories of Bain, Spencer, Carpenter, and Laycock in Britain.[37] However, unlike the British writers from which he derived his basic approach to the emotions, as a medical psychologist Maudsley was primarily concerned with the pathological aspects of mental phenomena. He was keen to stress the importance of establishing a solid theoretical foundation for his profession, and used his rising status in British psychological medicine to work towards this end. Danziger suggests that '[w]hen Maudsley became editor of the *Journal of Mental Science* in 1862, its scope began to broaden to include relevant theoretical articles of a psychological or even philosophical nature'.[38] His writings on mind and brain were at the core of the formation of British medical psychology as a scientific discipline concerned with empirical research into the causes, classification, and treatment of mental disease. Maudsley's physiological approach to mental pathology remained largely consistent throughout a career spanning more than four decades, but his nosology of insanity underwent several significant revisions. Key to these changes was that melancholia received increasingly more attention in his later work. His conceptualisation of melancholia rested upon a macro-classification developed early on in his published work that remained in place despite later nosological restructurings, and which saw mental disease divided into two umbrella categories: affective and ideational insanity.

Maudsley's framework for explaining mental phenomena was constructed around two related principles: reflex action, and organism–environment interaction, with the former occurring as a result of the latter. Maudsley perceived reflex action to be the most basic function of the nervous system. Like Griesinger, Laycock, and Carpenter, he did not reserve automated reactions only for unconscious bodily function. Rather, reflexive action developed in an evolutionary fashion and served as the core mechanism behind conscious thought as well as emotion. In basic terms, Maudsley perceived reflexion as the 'relation between the individual organism and the external nature', a process which could become progressively more complex, and in its higher forms was understood as 'sensory perception' and 'sensorimotor reaction'.[39] Drawing on ideas about environment–organism interaction developed by British psychologist Herbert Spencer in the 1850s, Maudsley suggested that a state of equilibrium between the external and the internal was at the core of all cerebral, and consequently all mental, functions. This was key to understanding the difference between normal and pathological emotionality:

> Certainly [the nerve cells] are not inexhaustible centres of self-generating force; they give out no more than what they have in one way or another taken in; they receive material from the blood, which they assimilate, or make of the same *kind* with themselves; a correlative metamorphosis of force necessarily accompanying this upward transformation of matter, and the nerve cells thus becoming, so long as its equilibrium is preserved, a centre of statical power of the highest vital quality.[40]

This 'statical power' can be compared to Griesinger's 'tone' discussed above. Perceived by Maudsley as 'the condition of latent thought', of a mind at rest, it constituted the epitome of psychological health. Equilibrium was thus both a physiological principle of 'self-regulation' as well as a mental state. When perfect balance was maintained, the mind was in a state of rest—of 'latent thought'. Following from this, 'the manifestation of thought' could be understood as 'the change or destruction of nervous element'.[41] Such a 'change or destruction' would be caused by a stimulus triggering a reaction. Following Griesinger, Maudsley held that such stimuli need not come from outside, but could equally have their origin somewhere in the body. Interaction, then, was also an intra-organism process. Equally, Maudsley perceived, like Laycock and Griesinger, a type of non-motor reflex action occurring within the brain resulting in ideas or emotional reactions rather than muscle contraction.[42] And like Griesinger, Maudsley suggested that emotional and ideational reactions to internal or external stimuli could occur without conscious awareness, producing a feeling of which the individual would not know the source, meaning it was prone to result in 'illusions with regard to the cause'. Such illusions often constituted symptoms of insanity, and were most frequently seen in asylum patients, he argued.[43]

In Maudsley's model of the mind the gradual development of consciousness, both within each individual and in an entire species across time, began as a reflexive relationship between environment and organism, where the former would act upon the latter, causing a corresponding reaction and, subsequently, transformation. In higher animals, this reflexive relationship formed the basis of the creation of new ideas. Like Griesinger, he suggested that impressions received by the brain would disperse internally and turn into 'ideas or conceptions', which could be 'pleasurable or painful, or have other particularly *emotional* qualities'.[44] As suggested above, Maudsley also followed Griesinger in arguing that psychological reflex action could occur both subconsciously and involuntarily; however, involuntary mental reflex action could also take place with the consciousness alerted yet 'in direct defiance of volitional effort'.[45] In the same manner as ideas and emotions the will was, according to Maudsley, the product of 'molecular change in a definitively constituted nervous centre', meaning that volition was, ultimately, 'excited into activity by the appropriate stimulus'.[46]

For Maudsley, then, volition did not belong to a higher realm independent from thought and emotion, it was a function of human biology, a physiological reaction to stimulus, if one that could be honed through persistent practice to function in a certain way. Not everyone who submitted to a physiological theory of mind was equally prepared to do away with the concept of free will. As discussed in Chapter 2, Carpenter divided the nervous system into hierarchically organised sections, with the intellect (containing the will) belonging to the highest sphere and immune from automated reaction. When describing psychological as opposed to sensory-motor reflex action, Maudsley deployed Carpenter's term 'ideo-motor' action, denoting its function as analogous to sensory-motor action. In Carpenter's original use of this term the principle extended as far as 'emotions' and 'instincts', and in some instances also 'ideas', but when it came to volition he would not concede to a reduction of the will to physiological processes.

When Maudsley used Carpenter's 'ideo-motor action', then, he also subtly changed its meaning. For Maudsley, all reactions of the mind were essentially equal. This meant that emotion was a reaction of the cerebral hemispheres just like volition and ideation (cognition). However, Maudsley differentiated emotion in other ways. Recalling his earlier remarks about a state of mental harmony, emotional reactions were for Maudsley what ensued in response to any form of imbalance, or unequal relationship, between the individual and their environment:

> As long as the ideas or mental states are not adequately organized in correspondence with the individual's external relations, more or less feeling will attend their excitation; they will, in fact, be more or less emotional. When the equilibrium between the subjective and objective is duly established, there is no passion, and there is but little emotion.[47]

Since any mental reactions could be triggered by external and internal stimuli alike, this was also the case for the emergence of pathological emotionality. In describing the process by which emotion would arise Maudsley stated that '[t]he equilibrium between the individual and his surroundings may, in fact, be disturbed by a subjective modification, or an internal commotion, as well as by an unwonted impression from without'.[48] The environment could act upon the individual, but so could the individual's own bodily operations, which in turn had the ability to affect the external–internal balance.

The kind of internal commotion described above would generally consist in some form of 'derangement' elsewhere in the body. This would then affect the brain, resulting in cerebral morbidity. Once this state had been reached, virtually any impression, including those that would trigger feelings of pleasure in a mind free from disease, would cause painful emotions.[49] This mental pain was made into a coherent medical phenomenon through being analogous to physical pain. This was the state that would prevail when the equilibrium of the mind was permanently upset, or, rather, when the 'tone' was disturbed. There is no reference to Griesinger here, but Maudsley's description of how morbid ideas and emotions emerge strongly echoes that of the German psychiatrist. The kinds of mental reactions that were likely to occur in response external or internal stimuli would depend on the '*psychical* tone, the tone of the supreme nervous centres', which was different in each individual as it was the long-term product of 'past thoughts, feelings, and actions, which have been organised as mental faculties'.[50]

While emotional reactions were produced in the brain, they would, through the various nervous connections of the human body, exert influence over bodily functions and trigger reactions of 'the organic movements, or the more intimate processes of nutrition'.[51] Emotion as physiological mental reflex action was a two-way process, in that it could be set off by some activity elsewhere in the body which would affect the brain and produce emotion, the latter which would then effect some other peripheral reaction (for instance, trembling). Moreover, yet another reciprocal action would occur from this: any emotion 'is rendered stronger and more distinct by the existence of those bodily states which it naturally produces'.[52] Cerebral and somatic reactions, both of which featured in the production of emotions, were mutually constitutive and reinforcing, maintaining the emotional state produced.[53] This process was particularly significant in the case of morbid emotional activity:

> Consequently, it is found that, as the effect of the depressing passion is felt by the victim of a local idiosyncrasy in his weak organ, so inversely the effect of a weak or diseased organ is felt in the brain by an irritability or disposition to passion, a disturbance of the psychical tone. The phenomena of insanity will furnish the best illustrations of this sympathetic interaction.[54]

Towards a Nosological Reification of Melancholia

According to Maudsley, not all individuals were equally prone to insanity. While morbid states may at times appear to be produced by a particular event or sudden 'mental shock', this would only be the immediate triggering factor. The conditions of mental disturbance consisted in an accumulation of physical and psychological factors over time, thus the cause of mental disease could be correctly discerned by means of '[a] complete biographical account of the individual'.[55] The process whereby the conditions of mental disease were gradually developed in a person was dependent upon the individual's capacity for adaptation. In conclusion, then, the aetiology of mental disease was for Maudsley ultimately a product of evolutionary law, where a healthy mind was 'the consequence and evidence of a successful adaptation to the conditions of existence', whereas mental disorder signified 'a failure in organic adaptation to external conditions', leading to 'disorder, decay, and death'.[56]

Such 'disorder, decay, and death' would in most cases begin with affective disturbance. Because disordered emotion could, in Maudsley's view, manifest without intellectual delusion, he rejected 'the present artificial classification, which is not really in conformity with nature'.[57] This classification or (various, similar) classifications which Maudsley referred to were commonly the product of cumulated models of some of the most often cited European alienists of the early nineteenth century, specifically Pinel, Esquirol, Guislain, and Griesinger. The major standard British textbook at the time, Tuke and Bucknill's *Manual of Psychological Medicine*,[58] adopted a nosology broadly based chiefly on Griesinger and Esquirol. In particular 'monomania', a British version of Esquirol's disease concept, served as an umbrella category for a number of sub-syndromes. These were considered various forms of 'partial' insanity, in other words disorders where some part of the power of intellectual reasoning was preserved.

As discussed in Chapter 3, the French physician's 'monomania' had been primarily defined as insanity relating to one specific object.[59] This category, and the many modifications of it, allowed for madness to be chiefly of emotional character, with only part of the intellect affected. However, it did not categorically distinguish between madness with or without delusion. In the 1858 edition of Bucknill and Tuke's textbook, melancholia was subsumed under 'monomania', though the authors recognised a version of it presenting 'without delusion'.[60] A separate category, 'emotional insanity', did not include forms of melancholia but rather chiefly mania and various forms of morbid impulsivity such as the 'homicidal impulse'. In sum, forms of madness where some form of ideational derangement was present.[61] Such a system of classification was, however, construed around an 'artificial exactness', Maudsley argued, and did not correspond to the endless plurality and complexity of mental disease. Would a nosological system not be more 'scientific', he asked, '[i]f a broad division was made of insanity into two classes, namely, insanity without positive delusion and insanity with delusion, in other words, into affective insanity and ideational insanity; and if the subdivision of these into varieties were subsequently made'?[62] The nosology Maudsley presented, then, insisted upon a marked division between mental disorders where partial or complete delusion was present, and illness where only the emotions were affected (Table 4.1).

One significant consequence of this division was that melancholia did not appear as a single, unified disease category. It was not primarily defined and organised according to its specific symptoms, but instead according to their source and character: that is, according to whether those symptoms consisted only in disordered emotion or in disordered ideation (or cognition) as well. Melancholia shared the category affective insanity with mania and with Maudsley's 'moral alienation', the latter which can be seen as one of the many variations of Prichard's moral insanity. The term 'moral' could mean either 'psychological' or moral as in ethical. Maudsley used it to mean the latter, a perversion of a person's moral character, resulting from a morbid emotional state. Maudsley's nosology was foundational for the idea of melancholia as a biomedical disorder of the emotions, since it unambiguously established as a medical principle the concept of pathological mood without concomitant intellectual derangement. This chapter and Chapter 2 showed how Laycock and Griesinger developed mental reflex models which allowed for the idea of pathological emotions, and how the latter stressed the role of the

Table 4.1 Classification of insanity (*The Physiology and Pathology of the Mind*, 1867)

Affective insanity	Ideational insanity
1. Maniacal Perversion of the Affective Life. Mania sine Delerio	1. General Mania (acute & chronic) Melancholia (acute & chronic)
2. Melancholic Depression without Delusion. Simple Melancholia	2. Partial Monomania Melancholia
3. Moral Alienation Proper	3. Dementia (primary & secondary)
	4. General Paralysis
	5. Idiocy (incl. Imbecility)

emotions as the key to understanding the emergence and progression of mental disease, arguing that all forms of insanity began with disordered emotions and mental pain. With Maudsley's nosology, disordered mood was unequivocally cemented as a specific, distinct form of mental disorder.

Maudsley was aware of the significance and implications of his system of classification; indeed, its implications for the diagnosis, treatment, and future research into insanity were his motivation for presenting it. Any nosology that did not fully and clearly recognise that a person could be gravely disturbed without being delusional was highly problematic, even dangerous. 'To insist upon the existence of delusion as a criterion of insanity', Maudsley argued, 'is to ignore some of the gravest and most dangerous forms of mental disease.' As discussed above, when the brain would begin to produce morbid emotions, these would become all-consuming, further entrenching the conflict between the internal and external life which was at the core of this disordered process as well as of healthy emotional reactions. Since this process occurred reflexively, analogous to automatic sensory-motor action, it was beyond the control of volition. To sum up, then,

> when there is perversion of the affective life, there will be morbid feeling and morbid action; the patient's whole manner of feeling, the mode of his affection by events, is unnatural, and the springs of his action are disordered; and the intellect is unable to check or control the morbid manifestations, just as, when there is disease of the spinal cord, there may be convulsive movement, of which there is consciousness, but which the will cannot restrain.[63]

Yet, this total engulfment of the individual by mental pain could take place without distorting the intellect. In the decades that followed a number of physicians, including Maudsley himself, would argue that it was this very feature which made the emotional pain of melancholia so difficult for sufferers to bear, and as such was a crucial factor in driving melancholics to suicide.

MELANCHOLIA ON THE CONTINENT: *FOLIE CIRCULAIRE* AND *PSYCHISCHE NEURALGIE*

The nosological status of melancholia was also being renegotiated on the continent in the mid-to-late nineteenth century. As shown in Chapter 3, Esquirol had proposed *lypemanie* as a replacement category for melancholia, indicating that it was a subspecies of monomania. The term never took off, but in the 1850s one of his protégés, Jules Baillarger, offered a more durable reconceptualisation of melancholia. Medical writers across Europe had occasionally suggested that the symptoms of melancholia could in some cases pass into those of mania and back again. For Baillarger, this oscillating process constituted a variety of madness, which he described in a paper read at the Imperial Academy of Medicine in Paris in 1854, and which was translated for an English-speaking audience the same year. Baillarger argued that while the two conditions appeared so much each other's opposites as to be 'strangers to each other', on the contrary, 'in most cases melancholia follows mania, and vice versa, as if there were a secret union between these two diseases'.[64] A similar proposition had, apparently unbeknownst to Baillarger, been made in a published article three years previously by fellow alienist Jean-Pierre Falret, who in response to Baillarger's paper remarked that he had been observing this form of mental derangement for some time on asylum wards, and had concluded that it was not merely 'a variety, but a specific form of insanity'. Falret had named this condition *folie circulaire*—circular insanity. He viewed it as a more or less lifelong, chronic illness, but with milder symptoms than were often found in melancholia and mania proper.[65]

The apparent discovery of this new disease was noted in Britain and was often referred to in discussions of melancholia in the decades that followed. While it was never widely appropriated in Victorian medical literature, British writers told of similar observations among asylum patients. Maudsley, for instance, suggested that melancholic symptoms could sometimes be a precursor to mania, and were prone to return again during the convalescent phase of the disease.[66] Thomas Clouston noted the presence of a form of mental disease that had 'been called by the French "circular insanity"', but suggested that a more appropriate term was that of 'alternating insanity', as in his view this type of madness was marked by distinctive changes in the person's overall character. 'Such men have three distinct lives', he argued, 'each of which is characterised by its own tastes, habits, dispositions, and modes of intellectual activity'.[67] George Savage remarked in a discussion on mania that a form of illness referred to as *folie circulaire* had been observed, in which 'mania is succeeded by melancholia, to be again succeeded either by a period of health, or by a fresh attack of mania.'[68] However, Savage held such cases to be 'extremely rare' among English lunatics, suggesting that in most of the patients under his care who had exhibited such a circular symptom picture, the proper diagnosis was one of 'recurrent mania', sometimes ending in dementia.[69] This statement largely reflected the view of his peers; while some writers used the term 'circular insanity' or *folie circulaire*, it was predominantly to talk of a subvariety of melancholia or mania.[70]

If the French model of circular insanity failed to gain widespread theoretical popularity or practical use in Britain at the time, German late nineteenth-century conceptions of melancholia were more extensively appropriated. By the mid-1870s, psychiatry was an established academic discipline across German-speaking Europe, particularly in former Prussia. Proponents of the new, scientific psychiatry were keen to define their work in opposition to the more traditional asylum-focused alienism, where both clinical practices and theoretical discussions had been chiefly aimed at management and confinement of lunatics. There was a strong focus on diagnostics, treatment, and clinical instruction for medical students of mental disease, and the discipline had from the start assumed a heavy leaning towards neurological conceptions of madness. As noted above, Griesinger had prior to his untimely death been a driving force in the early stages of this process, aptly symbolised by his appointment to the first combined chair in psychiatry and neurology at the Charité in Berlin in 1865.[71] However, Griesinger's model of melancholia remained partly wedded to traditional ideas; he maintained the old tripartite division of insanity, and while melancholia was fashioned with a modern, biomedical explanatory model, the symptom picture was little changed from that found in the works of earlier writers. While highlighting the modern 'mental depression' as a defining symptom, grief, despondency, and sadness were also primary features of Griesinger's melancholia, and he placed significant focus on the patient's overall constitution, physiognomy, and temperament. There was, moreover, little talk of suicidality.[72]

Less than a decade after Griesinger's death, in 1874, Austrian neurologist and psychiatrist Richard von Krafft-Ebing published a short monograph entitled *Die Melancholie: Eine Klinische Studie*. Krafft-Ebing would later become famous across Europe for his widely appropriated work on sexual pathology; however, his impressive catalogue of publications also included a comprehensive general textbook on mental disease aimed at students and practitioners, which appeared in several editions.[73] While the monograph on melancholia was never translated into English, significant parts of it were later absorbed into the English language version of his textbook on insanity, thus reaching a wider audience in Britain.[74] Krafft-Ebing's approach to emotion can be seen as closely aligned with Laycock's and Griesinger's. Emotion was a neurophysiological reaction analogous to action elsewhere in the body. In this way, melancholia was for Krafft-Ebing a form of 'mental neuralgia' (*psychische Neuralgie*), which was functionally different from physical neuralgia. The latter took the form of a 'bodily pain' along the 'sensory paths' of nervous transmission. In its psychological equivalent the brain was the object of 'excitement', producing 'an alteration of consciousness' manifesting as 'mental (*geistiger*) pain, a feeling which finds its expression through a change in mood'.[75] This psychic pain defined and dominated the overall mental state of the melancholic, and arose from internal rather than external causes.

Similar to Griesinger's model, this painful state of mind in Krafft-Ebing's melancholia was the result of repeated irritation of the brain. Mental neuralgia characterised the early stage of the illness, at which point neither the physiological process nor external symptoms were necessarily qualitatively different from those of a healthy mind. It follows that someone not trained in the skill of detecting mental disease would look for and expect to find the real cause of the mental pain. Here, however, lied the distinction between ordinary suffering and the suffering of simple, or non-delusional melancholia: the latter must be understood as an abnormal reaction to normal circumstances. Following Griesinger, Krafft-Ebing held that the melancholic brain would 'overreact' to external stimuli, so that all events, even those that would normally be a source of happiness, produced painful emotions.[76] 'Under such circumstances', he suggested, the origin of the mental pain 'is not psychic, but organic. It is the expression of a disturbance of nutrition in the psychic organ'.[77] In this pathological state, painful emotions would become self-perpetuating, with every impression brought upon the sick person becoming a source of further pain. Even the kinds of 'distractions' that would normally have a soothing or comforting influence, such as religion, would only produce further agony. Eventually the melancholic would reach a state where they were 'unable to rejoice over anything, but...equally unable to experience sadness'.[78]

Krafft-Ebing's work, then, contains one of the earliest descriptions of melancholia as a mental state characterised not by excessive low mood, but rather by an *absence* of feeling. Profound melancholia was, he argued, characterised by a lack of emotion—the patient becoming 'feeling-less' (*Gefühllos*) and 'mood-less' (*Gemühtlos*). This state of emotional apathy would often become so intolerable that the melancholic sufferer would eventually be driven to take their own life, prompting Krafft-Ebing to suggest that '[t]he majority of people who commit suicide are melancholics'. As will be seen in the next chapter, this perceived suicidality of melancholics placed a significant burden and responsibility on asylum staff, as such patients had to be kept under constant surveillance. In Krafft-Ebing's words, '[t]he cunning and perseverance exhibited by such sick people in the pursuit of their suicidal intentions' was so 'remarkable' that even the 'straitjacket is no guarantee against suicide'.[79]

MOOD DISORDER OR NERVOUS EXHAUSTION? MELANCHOLIA AND NEURASTHENIA

Krafft-Ebing's melancholic would sink so deeply into despair that they would eventually lose the ability to feel anything at all, even sadness, a defining symptom of traditional melancholia. This kind of emotional apathy was equally characteristic of neurasthenia, or nervous exhaustion, a 'disease of civilisation' emerging in the second half of the nineteenth century. Melancholia and neurasthenia were two separate conditions, situated within different explanatory frameworks and with different symptomatologies. But much like in the present, diagnostic boundaries in the nineteenth century were often fuzzy and fluid, and the neurophysiological framework for explaining mental disease expounded by Griesinger, Maudsley, Krafft-Ebing, and others coexisted with a more general discourse on 'nerves' as a source of a wide variety of mental and physical symptoms for which no organic cause could be found. As one historian notes, much in the same way as 'an epileptic fit might be explained in terms of excessive build-up and then discharge of nervous energy, so the symptoms of depression, fatigue, melancholia, and nervous breakdown could be attributed to the ebbing of the same force'.[80] 'Mental depression' in particular, a symptom denoting a mind 'pressed down', served to bridge melancholia and neurasthenia, and have led scholars to discuss nineteenth-century experiences of low mood, fatigue, sadness, inertia, anxiety, and despair under the general heading of 'depression'.[81]

While it is not possible to fully disentangle the two conditions from each other, it is important to note their clear differences as well as their similarities. Neurasthenia emerged in the United States in the 1860s. E.H. van Deusen and George Beard are both credited with coining the term, but the latter is generally regarded as its chief proponent. The symptoms of neurasthenia as described by Beard in his famous monograph on the condition tell of a diffuse and all-encompassing illness, a mental and bodily malaise that left few parts of the human anatomy untouched. Sufferers of this disease would, according to Beard, complain of a diverse assortment of symptoms, including headaches, tenderness of the scalp, digestive problems, visual disturbances, noises in the ears, cramps, heart palpitations, back pain, dry skin, tenderness of the teeth and gums, insomnia, drowsiness, mental irritability, hopelessness, and morbid fear.[82] Misbach and Stam suggest that neurasthenia was seen by some as a more attractive diagnosis as it was predominantly conceptualised as a somatic condition rather than a mental disorder, and therefore came with less stigma attached.[83] This made it particularly popular with the upper classes, and to the extent the diagnosis was deployed in Europe this was primarily in the context of private practices rather than on asylum wards.

Much like the language around emotion, the discourse on nerves that underpinned neurasthenia underwent a reconceptualisation in the nineteenth century. The idea of 'nerves' as the cause and manifestation of poor mental and physical health had been popular in early modern Britain, and was famously discussed at length by eighteenth-century physician George Cheyne in his treatise on 'the English malady'.[84] The eighteenth-century explanatory framework was, however, different from that of the following century, the former attributing nervous suffering to 'weak, loose, and feeble or relaxed nerves',[85] suggesting that this was a problem primarily affecting the higher social strata whose way of life had made them particularly sensitive. Weak nerves were linked to 'the high-living, prosperity, and progress unique on such a wide scale in eighteenth-century England'.[86] From the mid-nineteenth century onward, however, nervous disorders became explicitly understood as *exhaustion* resulting not from affluent living, but from the increasing pressures of 'brain work' in a rapidly expanding capitalist society.[87] Moreover, it was no longer the loss of vital fluid that was the main source of disease, but rather the loss of 'force'.[88] As Anson Rabinbach has shown, the human body became metaphorically perceived as an engine subject to the same laws as heat powered machinery.[89] This new way of conceptualising health and sickness borrowed its language and explanatory model from the theory of thermodynamics, which merged with terminology derived from economics. The increasing popularity of the word depression as a medical symptom must be understood in the context of these developments, which highlight the role of this symptom in blurring the line between emotional disorders such as melancholia and the more somatically framed concept of nervous exhaustion. In this context the word 'depression' became a more frequent and prominent part of medical terminology, specifically in regards to mental states.[90] The growing popularity of this word as a feature both of nervous exhaustion and medical melancholy can no doubt in part account for the tendency among contemporary scholars to equate nineteenth-century nervous conditions as well as melancholia with 'depression' as understood in late twentieth- and twenty-first-century medical discourse.

Both melancholia and neurasthenia were somatically framed, and both were unlikely to turn up structural organic evidence of disease. In this way, both conditions could be seen to straddle the increasingly fluid boundary between normal and pathological states, but while there was certainly some overlap between the two, it is crucial to note that they were fundamentally different conditions. Nervous exhaustion was brought about by external pressures, whereas melancholia was primarily the result of an internal pathology—though as we have seen, this mental state could be triggered by both internal and external factors, making the aetiology of melancholia ambiguous. Neurasthenia was a poorly defined, diffuse somatic condition whose validity was contested among many psychiatrists, whereas melancholia was a clearly demarcated mental disease with a coherent symptomatology centred on depressed mood, mental pain, and suicidality, and in the more severe stages of the illness inertia, bodily retardation, delusions and hallucinations, and in some cases catatonia. Melancholia was unequivocally perceived as a form of insanity. However, while neurasthenia is today an object of study for historians of psychiatry, its status in the late nineteenth century was less clear. It was originally conceptualised as a somatic condition, but towards the turn of the century as physicians had repeatedly failed to turn up organic evidence of disease, the symptoms were increasingly seen as 'functional'. As a consequence, the category moved into the realm of psychiatry, eventually becoming reconceptualised as 'neurosis' within the emergent psychoanalytical tradition.[91]

MELANCHOLIA ACROSS THE ATLANTIC

The complex relationship between melancholy and neurasthenia must also be understood with reference to geographical and cultural differences. The neurasthenia diagnosis never really took off in Europe's medical circles. Beard himself remarked that neurasthenia was far more common in North America than in Western Europe, highlighting a divergence between the two realms. Melancholia was deployed as a diagnosis in North-American asylums and US physicians published on the disease, but the diagnosis was primarily shaped and standardised through the works of British and German authors. Descriptions of the condition in North-American journals demonstrate the influence of European psychiatry on US conceptualisations of melancholia. In a lecture on melancholia delivered in 1876 Daniel Kitchen, head of New York's Blackwell Island asylum, endorsed a model of disordered mood anchored in physiological psychology. Echoing Griesinger, Kitchen noted that all forms of insanity began with disordered action of 'the emotional reflex centres'. Like Griesinger, he also appeared to subscribe to the unitary model of mental disease, referring to melancholia as the 'first stage' of insanity. Kitchen described the progression from simple, non-delusional melancholia to more severe forms, in which both delusions and hallucinations could develop. He also noted the prominence of suicidal tendencies, which, he argued, may cause patients to try to convince the physician that they were well enough to be released 'in order to obtain their object'. Kitchen's description of melancholia illustrates the extent to which the diagnosis was becoming standardised in the West in the second half of the century as a clearly defined condition with a largely coherent symptomatology. Indeed, Kitchen remarked that diagnosing melancholia was 'not difficult' as 'nearly all cases' were 'self-evident'.[92]

Ira Russell, writing for the *Alienist and Neurologist* in 1881, equally placed melancholia in a psycho-physiological framework. Drawing on the works of British physicians such as Tuke and Bucknill, Crichton Browne, and Maudsley, Russell suggested that '[m]orbid states...of the centres of organic sensation in reciprocal action and reaction may give rise to hypochondriasis or melancholia'.[93] He moreover strongly emphasised the importance of being vigilant towards suicidal propensities in melancholics, arguing that the 'tendency of melancholics to commit suicide, renders it absolutely necessary that they should be carefully watched.'[94] Here Russell echoed a claim forcefully made by Maudsley, Savage, and other British physicians of the period, as will be seen in the next chapter. In explaining the suicidality of melancholics he cited Maudsley, who 'says it is due to the loss of the love of life'. Speculating about the physiological basis for this deviation from what was at the time considered an evolutionary fact, Russell pondered whether there might 'be a cerebral center that presides over the instinctive love of life' and that in the case of suicidal melancholics 'that center' had become 'organically or functionally diseased'.[95]

CONCLUSION

By the last quarter of the century, a biomedical model of melancholia as a condition of disordered mood was widely endorsed across Western Europe and North America. This chapter has shown how Griesinger developed a theory of psychological reflex action similar to that put forward by Laycock, which he subsequently deployed to explain how emotion became disordered through repeated irritation of the brain, eventually resulting in pathology. This pathological mental state, which in the early stages would usually manifest as simple melancholia, or sometimes hypochondria, could deteriorate to the point where delusions and hallucinations developed. For Griesinger and some other contemporaneous writers, melancholia was the first in three stages of mental disease, meaning that if left untreated it was likely to progress into mania, and eventually dementia and death. Others, such as Maudsley, did not subscribe to the unitary psychosis model, conceiving instead of melancholia as a distinct illness category (or categories). These differences should not, however, be overstated. From the point of view of aetiology and diagnostics, the internal model and the symptomatology of melancholia were largely the same whether classified as an independent disease or as the first stage of insanity. Towards the end of the century, the diagnosis was increasingly standardised in published literature, where it came to centre on four key symptoms: mental pain, depression, suicidality, and religious delusions. This is the focus of the next chapter.

NOTES

1. Henry Maudsley, *The Physiology and Pathology of the Mind* (London: Macmillan, 1867), 302.

2. Gerlof Verwey offers an engaging account of Griesinger's life in *Wilhelm Griesinger: Psychiatrie als ärztlicher Humanismus* (Nijmegen: Arts & Boeve, 2004).

3. See Wilhelm Griesinger, "The Care and Treatment of the Insane in Germany," *Journal of Mental Science* 14, No. 65 (1868): 1–34. The original article, which caused a stir among his German peers, was published in the introductory issue of the *Archiv für Psychiatrie und Nervenkrankheiten*, which Griesinger launched together with Ludwig Meyer and Carl Westphal in 1867. For the events leading to the creation of this journal (which sought to distance itself from the more traditional asylum journals), see Alexander Mette, *Wilhelm Griesinger: Der Begründer der Wissenschaftligen Psychiatrie in Deutschland* (Leipzig: Teubner, 1976), 58–67. For more detailed commentary/discussions of Griesinger's reform program see: Eric J. Engstrom, *Clinical Psychiatry in Imperial Germany: A History of Psychiatric Practice* (Ithaca, NY: Cornell University Press, 2004), 51–87; Kai Sammet, "'Ueber Irrenanstalten und deren Weiterentwicklung in Deutschland': Wilhelm Griesinger im Streit mit der konservativen Anstaltspsychiatrie 1865–1868" (PhD diss., Hamburg, Münster, 2000).

4. Wilhelm Griesinger, "Ueber psychische Reflexactionen: Mit einem Blick auf das Wesen der psychischen Krankheiten," reprinted in *Gesammelte Abhandlungen, Ersters Band: Psychiatrische Abhandlungen* (Amsterdam: E.J. Bonset, 1968 [1843]).

5. Griesinger, "Ueber psychische Reflexactionem," 4–5.

6. Griesinger, "Ueber psychische Reflexactionem," 11–12.

7. Edward Shorter, *A History of Psychiatry: From the Era of the Asylum to the Age of Prozac* (New York: Wiley, 1997), 76.

8. Griesinger, "Ueber psychische Reflexactionem," 10–11.

9. Gerlof Verwey, *Psychiatry in an Anthropological and Biomedical Context: Philosophical Presuppositions and Implications of German Psychiatry, 1820–1870* (Dordrecht: Kluwer, 1985), 87.

10. Herbert Spencer, *The Principles of Psychology* (London: Longman, Brown, Green & Longmans, 1855).

11. Griesinger, Griesinger, "Ueber psychische Reflexactionem," 24–25, 35–36.

12. Griesinger, "Ueber psychische Reflexactionem," 35.

13. Wilhelm Griesinger, "The Prognosis in Mental Disease," *Journal of Mental Science* 11 (1865): 317–321.

14. Verwey suggests that Griesinger built his theory of unitary psychosis partly on his mentor Alfred Zeller's beliefs, and partly on the model developed by Belgian physician Joseph Guislain; Verwey, *Psychiatry*, 141–143. Guislain's psychiatric nosology was influential across Western Europe in the first half of the century. See Joseph Guislain, *Traité sur l'Aliénation Mentale et sur les Hospices des Aliénalés* (Amsterdam: J. van der Hey, 1826). Despite the moderate popularity of some of his ideas, which were frequently cited by mid-century British physicians, there exist to my knowledge no English translations of his work. His treatise on mental disease was, however, translated into German in the 1850s.

15. Wilhelm Griesinger, *Die Pathologie und Therapie der psychischen Krankheiten*, 2 Aufl. (Stuttgart: Adolf Krabbe, 1861), 213–275.

16. Griesinger, "The Prognosis in Mental Disease," 317–327.

17. When Griesinger introduced his reform plan he did so from a position of moderate fame; his textbook and prestigious role at the Charité had made him well-known both in Germany and abroad. British readers were thus able to partake in Griesinger's vision for psychiatry when the speech that first made it public was translated into English and published in the *Journal of Mental Science* the following year. Griesinger, "Care and Treatment of the Insane."

18. German E. Berrios, *The History of Mental Symptoms: Descriptive Psychopathology since the Nineteenth Century* (Cambridge: Cambridge University Press, 1995), 310.

19. Griesinger, *Die Pathologie und Therapie*. For Zeller's influence on Griesinger see Verwey, *Psychiatry*, 140–150.

20. Griesinger, *Die Pathologie und Therapie*, 1.

21. This kind of physiological conception of mind potentially foreclosed the possibility of 'free will', since it made volition subject to the same abstract reflexive action as emotion. On free will in late-Victorian thought, see Roger Smith, *Free Will and the Human Sciences in Britain, 1870–1910* (London: Pickering and Chatto, 2013). It should be noted that eighteenth-century writers on the philosophy of mind, particularly Locke and Hume, discussed the interplay between the passions, ideas, and volition in ways that could also be read as suggesting no significant hierarchical distinction between these faculties. Nevertheless, such claims occurred within a framework of an abstract philosophical conception of mind; to conceive of emotions, ideas, and the will as similar, and equal, physiological operations of the brain have arguably had far greater consequences for perceptions of mental pathology in the modern period.

22. Griesinger, *Die Pathologie und Therapie*, 25.

23. Maudsley's nosology of 1867 was one of the first to put forward a type of madness in which the emotions were the only part of the mind affected, dividing thus the milder forms of insanity into 'affective' and 'ideational'.
24. Griesinger, *Die Pathologie und Therapie*, 26.
25. Griesinger, *Die Pathologie und Therapie*, 32.
26. Griesinger, *Die Pathologie und Therapie*, 33.
27. Griesinger, *Die Pathologie und Therapie*, 34.
28. Griesinger, *Die Pathologie und Therapie*, 213.
29. Griesinger, *Die Pathologie und Therapie*, 214.
30. Griesinger, *Die Pathologie und Therapie*, 215.
31. Griesinger, *Die Pathologie und Therapie*, 215–216.
32. Griesinger, *Die Pathologie und Therapie*, 227. For an account of the evolution of pain without organic injury, see Andrew Hodgkiss, *From Lesion to Metaphor: Chronic Pain in British, French and German Medical Writings, 1800–1914* (Amsterdam: Rodopi, 2000). Chapter 4, "Reflexion and Depression" discusses psychological reflex action according to Müller, Griesinger, and Laycock in relation to developments of ideas about 'pain without lesion'. Hodgkiss's book provides important historical context to current medical views regarding bodily 'symptoms' without apparent organic cause, and concurrent debates about 'psycho-somatic illness'.
33. Griesinger, *Die Pathologie und Therapie*, 228.
34. Cf. Maudsley on simple melancholia, Chapter 5.
35. Griesinger, *Die Pathologie und Therapie*, 228–229. As will be seen in Chapter 5, Maudsley developed this model of simple melancholia in more detail in the last decade of the century, arguing that the ability of simple melancholics to reason about their suffering meant that they were more likely to commit suicide than melancholics whose illness was so severe that they had developed delusional thinking.
36. Biographical accounts of Maudsley can be found in: Aubrey Lewis, "Henry Maudsley: His Work and Influence (25th Maudsley Lecture)," *Journal of Mental Science* 407 (1951): 260–277; Trevor Turner, "Henry Maudsley: Psychiatrist, Philosopher, and Entrepreneur," in *The Anatomy of Madness: Essays in the History of Psychiatry, Vol. III: The Asylum and Its Psychiatry*, eds. William F. Bynum, Roy Porter, and Michael Shepherd (London: Routledge, 1988), 151–187; Michael Collie, *Henry Maudsley: Victorian Psychiatrist: A Bibliographical Study* (Winchester: St Paul's Bibliographies, 1988). Maudsley has received particular attention for his views on sex and degeneration, see e.g. Elaine Showalter, *The Female Malady: Women, Madness, and English Culture, 1830–1980* (London: Virago, 1987); Daniel Pick, *Faces of Degeneration: A European Disorder, c. 1848–1918* (Cambridge: Cambridge University Press, 1989).
37. Maudsley, *Physiology and Pathology of the Mind*, 45.
38. Danziger, "British Psycho-Physiology," 138.

39. Maudsley, *Physiology and Pathology of the Mind*, 45.
40. Maudsley, *Physiology and Pathology of the Mind*, 41.
41. Maudsley, *Physiology and Pathology of the Mind*, 41–42.
42. Maudsley, *Physiology and Pathology of the Mind*, 88–89.
43. Maudsley, *Physiology and Pathology of the Mind*, 103.
44. Maudsley, *Physiology and Pathology of the Mind*, 47. Emphasis in original.
45. Maudsley, *Physiology and Pathology of the Mind*, 108.
46. Maudsley, *Physiology and Pathology of the Mind*, 149–150. For the will as physiological reflex, see also Henry Maudsley, *Body and Mind* (London: Macmillan, 1870), 27.
47. Maudsley, *Physiology and Pathology of the Mind*, 129. While in a very general sense, the terms 'passions' and 'emotions' could be seen to constitute a traditional and a modern category respectively, they were used differently by different writers at the time, sometimes the two were deployed synonymously, sometimes to denote different feeling states (see Dixon, *From Passions to Emotions*). Taking note of this conundrum, Maudsley clarified his own usage: 'It may be thought, perhaps, that it would not be amiss if something were now said of the difference between passion and emotion, inasmuch as the terms have hitherto been used almost indifferently. This, however, is scarcely necessary in dealing only with their general nature, which is fundamentally the same; every so-called emotion, when carried to a certain pitch, becomes a veritable passion' (p. 141).
48. Maudsley, *Physiology and Pathology of the Mind*, 134–135.
49. Maudsley, *Physiology and Pathology of the Mind*, 135.
50. Maudsley, *Physiology and Pathology of the Mind*, 137. Emphasis in original.
51. Maudsley, *Physiology and Pathology of the Mind*, 139.
52. Maudsley, *Physiology and Pathology of the Mind*, 140.
53. On emotion and its bodily manifestations, cf. Alexander Bain and William James, respectively, for two related but importantly different models. For Bain, the physical reactions accompanying different feelings were central to the problem of the tension between emotion and volition. While Bain argued, as did Maudsley, that emotions could be successfully regulated or supressed through habit, he was primarily concerned with those bodily manifestations of emotion which he considered to be 'voluntary', such as gestures and facial expressions (to be contrasted with 'involuntary' reactions like blushing) rather than with the feelings themselves. Alexander Bain, *The Emotions and the Will* (London: John W. Parker and Son, 1859), esp. 398–402. For James, the bodily manifestations were the starting point, i.e. these reactions came first, and would consequently produce the psychological feeling. William James, "What Is an Emotion," *Mind* 9 (1884): 189–190.
54. Maudsley, *Physiology and Pathology of the Mind*, 141.

55. Maudsley, *Physiology and Pathology of the Mind*, 197. The practice of taking a person's medical 'history' was becoming standard practice in the mid-to-late nineteenth century. This development was gradually aided by the introduction of medical certificates, which explicitly asked medical officers to provide background information about new patients such as 'previous attacks', 'hereditary history', 'pre-disposing causes', and 'exciting (or immediate) causes'.
56. Maudsley, *Physiology and Pathology of the Mind*, 199.
57. Maudsley, *Physiology and Pathology of the Mind*, 322.
58. Which appeared in numerous editions over several decades.
59. Jean-Étienne Dominique Esquirol, *Mental Maladies: A Treatise on Insanity* (Philadelphia: Lea & Blanchard, 1845 [1838]), 209.
60. Bucknill and Tuke, *A Manual of Psychological Medicine*, 152, 181.
61. Bucknill and Tuke, *A Manual of Psychological Medicine*, 181–194.
62. Maudsley, *Physiology and Pathology of the Mind*, 322.
63. Maudsley, *Physiology and Pathology of the Mind*, 302.
64. (Author unknown) "Baillarger and Falret on a new species of insanity. Remarks on a variety of insanity, the paroxysms of which are characterized by two regular periods, the one of depression and the other of excitement by Dr. Baillarger," *The American Journal of Insanity* 11, No. 3 (1854–55): 230.
65. "Baillarger and Falret," 234. See also Jean-Pierre Falret, "De la folie circulaire ou forme de maladie mentale characterisée par L'alternative réguliere de la manie et de la mélancolie," *Bulletin de L'Academie Nationale de Médicine*, Paris (1851); German E. Berrios, "Melancholia and Depression during the Nineteenth Century: A Conceptual History," *British Journal of Psychiatry* 153 (1988): 301–302.
66. Maudsley, *The Pathology of Mind*, 382.
67. Thomas S. Clouston, "Report of the Physician-Superintendent for the Year 1881," *Annual Report for the Royal Edinburgh Asylum for the Insane*, Morningside, Royal Edinburgh Asylum (1882), 14. Maudsley later expressed a view closer to Clouston's, suggesting that in the '*folie circulaire* of French authors the person is as unlike in thought, feeling and conduct as two persons of different character'. Henry Maudsley, "The Physical Conditions of Consciousness," *Mind* 2, No. 48 (1887): 506.
68. Savage, *Insanity and Allied Neuroses*, 122.
69. Savage, *Insanity and Allied Neuroses*, 123. For other contemporary views on circular insanity in British asylum patients, see e.g. Bucknill and Tuke, *Manual of Psychological Medicine*, 4th ed., 137–138, 304; Sankey, "On Melancholia," 191; D.G. Thomson, "The Prognosis in Insanity," *Journal of Mental Science* 29 (1883): 194–195; W. Herbert Packer, "A Case of Circular Insanity (Folie Circulaire)," *Journal of Mental Science* 30 (1884): 62–64.

70. Savage's remark that circular insanity was unusual among British lunatics reveals little about different experiences of national asylum populations, and much about domestic coherence in knowledge and practices. Callard makes a similar remark in regards to Carl Westphal's model of agoraphobia, suggesting that presentations of 'remarkably similar symptomatologies need not be read as an empirical proof of how individuals in different countries were presenting with identical agoraphobic symptoms. Rather, those similarities could point to how potent Westphal's initial account was in providing compelling tropes and vignettes that were taken up elsewhere.' Felicity Callard, "'The Sensation of Infinite Vastness'; Or, the Emergence of Agoraphobia in the Late 19th Century," *Environment and Planning D: Society and Space* 24 (2006): 878.

71. See Engstrom, *Clinical Psychiatry*.

72. Griesinger, *Die Pathologie und Therapie*, 213.

73. Richard von Krafft-Ebing, *Lehrbuch der Psychiatrie auf klinischer Grundlag: für practische Ärzte und Studirende* (Stuttgart: Ferdinand Enke, 1880–1897).

74. Richard von Krafft-Ebing, *A Text-Book of Insanity Based on Clinical Observations* (New York: Classics of Psychiatry & Behavioral Sciences Library, 1992).

75. Richard von Krafft-Ebing, *Die Melancholie: Eine klinische Studie* (Erlangen: Ferdinand Enke, 1874), 1–4, 6. Mental pain as a symptom of melancholia is further discussed in Chapter 5.

76. Krafft-Ebing, *Melancholie*, 3–6, 9–11.

77. Krafft-Ebing, *Textbook of Insanity*, 49.

78. Krafft-Ebing, *Melancholie*, 5.

79. Krafft-Ebing, *Melancholie*, 65.

80. Roy Porter, "Nervousness, Eighteenth and Nineteenth Century Style: From Luxury to Labour," in *Cultures of Neurasthenia from Beard to the First World War*, ed. Marijke Gijswijt-Hofstra (Amsterdam and New York: Rodopi, 2001), 38.

81. Janet Oppenheim, *'Shattered Nerves': Doctors, Patients, and Depression in Victorian England* (Oxford: Oxford University Press, 1991).

82. George Beard, *A Practical Treatise on Nervous Exhaustion (Neurasthenia), Its Symptoms, Nature, Sequences, Treatment* (New York: William Wood, 1880), 15–69.

83. Judith Misbach and Henderikus J. Stam, "Medicalizing Melancholia: Exploring Profiles of Psychiatric Professionalization," *Journal of the History of the Behavioral Sciences* 42, No. 1 (2006): 41–59.

84. George Cheyne, *The English Malady, Or, A Treatise of Nervous Diseases of All Kinds, as Spleen, Vapour, Lowness of Spirits, Hypochondriacal or Hysterical Distempers* (London: George Strahan, 1733).

85. William F. Bynum, "The Nervous Patient in Eighteenth- and Nineteenth-Century Britain: The Psychiatric Origins of British Neurology," in *The Anatomy of Madness: Essays in the History of Psychiatry*, Vol. I: *People and Ideas*, eds. W.F. Bynum, Roy Porter, and Michael Shepherd (London: Routledge, 1985), 91. See also Porter, "Nervousness," 32–36.

86. Bynum, "The Nervous Patient," 91. This idea must moreover be placed in its wider medical context. Anne Vila has shown how weakness, strength, and vitality, inscribed onto nerves and tissue and linked to the body's 'vital fluids' (and both explicitly and implicitly gendered and moralised), accounted for unhealth more generally in the Enlightenment. Anne C. Vila, *Enlightenment and Pathology: Sensibility in the Literature and Medicine of Eighteenth-Century France* (Baltimore and London: The Johns Hopkins University Press, 1998), 65–73, 94–107, 229–240.

87. British medical accounts of nervous disorders abound in this period. See, for instance: (author unknown) "Nervous Influence," *Journal of Psychological Medicine and Mental Pathology* 5 (1852): 221–229; Cyril Bennet, *The Modern Malady, or, Sufferers from "Nerves"* (London: Edward Arnold, 1890); Edward Jarvis, "The Overworked Mind," *Journal of Psychological Medicine and Mental Pathology* 5 (1852): 257–276; George Lefevre, "An Apology for the Nerves, Or Their Influence and Importance in Health and Disease," *Journal of Psychological Medicine and Mental Pathology* 2 (1849): 90–114; James Ross, *Handbook of the Diseases of the Nervous System* (London: J & A Churchill, 1885); Thomas Stretch Dowse, *On Brain and Nerve Exhaustion: 'Neurasthenia'* (London: Baillière, Tindall & Cox, 1880).

88. Porter, "Nervousness," 37.

89. Anson Rabinbach, *The Human Motor: Energy, Fatigue, and the Origins of Modernity* (Berkeley: University of California Press, 1992), 23–25, 121, 124–127.

90. Berrios, "Melancholia and Depression," 300–301.

91. Michael Neve, "Public Views of Neurasthenia: Britain 1880–1930," in *Cultures of Neurasthenia*, ed. Gijswijt-Hofstra, 154–157; Porter, "Nervousness, Eighteenth and Nineteenth Century Style," 42–43; Chandak Sengoopta, "'A Mob of Incoherent Symptoms?' Neurasthenia in British Medical Discourse, 1860–1920," in ed. Gijswijt-Hofstra, *Cultures of Neurasthenia*, 107–110; Thomson, "Neurasthenia in Britain," 84–90.

92. Daniel H. Kitchen, "Lectures on Insanity. Lecture II: Melancholia, Delivered at Charity Hospital, October and November 1876," *Ohio Medical and Surgical Journal* 2, No. 3 (1877): 237–256.

93. Ira Russell, "Melancholia," *The Alienist and Neurologist* 2 (1881): 201.

94. Russell, "Melancholia," 202.

95. Russell, "Melancholia," 205.

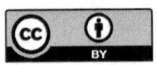

CHAPTER 5

Statistics, Classification, and the Standardisation of Melancholia

*No class of diseases with which man is afflicted are as various in their mani-
festations, as those known under the general term of insanity. No diseases
present such an infinite variety of light and shade belonging to their own
nature, or to their own intermixture with other maladies, or to the influence
of temperament, of individual peculiarities of habit, or of social position; and
therefore the diagnosis of no other class of diseases taxes nearly so much the
integrity and the patience of the physician.*[1]

John Charles Bucknill (1856)

*Classification is not the dry exercise of putting things into pigeonholes but the
act of creating the holes into which to put things.*[2]

Roger Smith (2007)

When Bethlem physician George Savage stated in the 1880s that '[a]ny
classification of insanity must necessarily be provisional',[3] he expressed
perhaps the one aspect of classification upon which most Victorian
alienists could agree. The classification of mental disease was a hotly
contested topic among nineteenth-century physicians—no standard,
universally accepted nosology existed, and diagnostic practices, labels,
and criteria could differ a great deal between different asylums and
hospitals. The British Lunacy Commission attempted to institute a
unified system with considerable success, but many physicians continued
to favour alternative nosologies, each often with their own idiosyncratic

© The Author(s) 2021   123
Å Jansson, *From Melancholia to Depression*,
Mental Health in Historical Perspective,
https://doi.org/10.1007/978-3-030-54802-5_5

twist. Biomedical models of mental disease dominated in the second half of the nineteenth century, and internal, physiological explanations for melancholia displayed notable coherence. However, such disease models were of little use when it came to diagnostics. While Savage and many of his peers expressed hope and confidence that it would one day become possible to identify and diagnose various forms of insanity according to 'the physiological changes which take place in the nerve centres',[4] they were presently guided in their diagnostic work by the presence or absence of external symptoms. Symptoms of melancholia were observed through the spectacles of physiology, and were shaped through biomedical language, giving prominence to 'depression' and 'mental pain', terms reconceptualised within a modern scientific framework. Another key symptom, 'religious delusions', emerged from patient interviews, which suggested that significant number of melancholics experienced their suffering as punishment from God. Finally, late-nineteenth-century physicians were in particular trained to look for 'suicidal tendencies' in melancholic patients, a problem believed to be so prevalent as to lead one physician to remark that '[t]he question of the patient being suicidal should never in any case of melancholia be left unconsidered, and the risk of his becoming suicidal should never in any case be left unprovided for'.[5]

The belief that a majority of melancholics were suicidal became something of an axiom for late-Victorian asylum physicians, and informed decisions about confinement, surveillance, and treatment of melancholic patients. The term itself emerged as a medical concept through the certificates of insanity that had to be filled out prior to a person's admission to the asylum, and which required a yes or no answer as to whether the suspected lunatic was 'epileptic, suicidal, or dangerous to others'.[6] This information was subsequently transferred into asylum admission records and casebooks, where it was entered alongside various other information about the patient, including the type of disease they were believed to suffer from. When statistics on suicidality were merged with diagnostic figures, these suggested that patients who entered the asylum with the label 'suicidal' on their certificate were far more likely to receive the diagnosis melancholia than other patients, leading to the assumption that all melancholics were potentially suicidal.[7]

Edwin Schneidman, a prominent twentieth-century British psychiatrist, wrote in 1993 that 'suicide is caused by *psychache*', a term he used to denote 'intolerable psychological pain'.[8] Perhaps unbeknownst to the author, this phrase echoes the words of nineteenth-century physicians who more than a century earlier suggested that melancholia was characterised by a 'psychic ache', 'mental pain', or 'psychalgia' that often led patients to become suicidal.[9] Schneidman's work has formed the basis for more recent research into the relationship between suicidality and mental pain.[10] In twenty-first-century psy-literature, the close relationship between these two phenomena is apparently taken for granted—intolerable mental pain produces suicidal thoughts and gestures, which sometimes lead to suicide. In the twenty-first century, 'depression'[11] conjures up similar anxieties about suicidality. Today the term is chiefly used in psychiatry to denote a specific condition—clinical depression or Major Depressive Disorder. The view that this condition carries a significant risk of suicide is accepted across Western medicine, and suicidality is listed as a diagnostic criterion of depression in the most recent editions of both the *DSM* and the *ICD*.[12] Much like the relationship between mental pain and suicidality, the causal bond between depression and suicidal thoughts and actions appears to be taken as self-evident in the present, in medical and non-medical contexts alike. In the Victorian period, there was no illness with this name, but the term was used with growing regularity, primarily to describe the overall mental and bodily state of the melancholic—a pressing down, a dulling of the individual's internal processes of 'nutrition'. Used in this way, the term denoted low mood, inertia, sluggishness, and a general slowing down of bodily functions such as respiration, digestion, speech, and, in some cases, even hair growth. Melancholia was often referred to in nosological literature as the 'state of mental depression',[13] contrasted with 'mental weakness' and 'exaltation'.

Religious delusions were frequently noted as a symptom of melancholia in case notes as well as published literature. Patients who arrived in the asylum and were diagnosed with melancholia commonly expressed profound feelings of guilt. Casebook descriptions tell of 'imaginary' sins committed, of desperate accounts of having 'caused the ruin of' and 'brought shame upon' one's family, of having done such horrible things that one was unworthy of life and must be punished by God. Such expressions of guilt and shame were noted by physicians as 'delusions' of a religious nature, a symptom of mental disease that contributed to melancholic patients' suicidal propensities. To the historian, this symptom illustrates the uneasy yet close relationship between old and new ideas, between spiritual and scientific worldviews and ways of experience. While it is not possible to access the 'true' experience of patients whose stories emerge only as case notes scribbled by their physicians, fears of God's punishment and of having brought shame upon one's family through sinful acts must be seen as very much real and present in what was, despite the arrival of modern science, still a largely Christian society, one that placed high value on 'virtues' such as respectability, godliness, purity, and self-help.[14]

As a symptom of melancholia, religious delusions have important contrasts with mental pain. The former were commonly described in case notes, admission documents, and published case studies, but were rarely held up as a defining criterion in textbook definitions of melancholia in the same way as the latter. Mental pain, conversely, was listed as a primary psychological symptom of melancholia in nosological descriptions, but was rarely used as an expressive term in asylum casebooks. From what can be deduced from patient records, it was not a word patients themselves used to talk about their suffering, however it did to some extent feature as a descriptive term in popular language. For Victorian physicians, its usefulness was chiefly as a unifying diagnostic term, a form of shorthand for a range of emotional expressions that asylum physicians took to be the manifestation of psychological pain. While the term itself had spiritual roots, as a medical symptom it was a distinctly modern one, presented in the literature as a physiological state analogous to physical pain.

The terms 'suicidal tendencies', 'depression', 'mental pain', and 'religious delusions' were produced as medical concepts in significantly different ways, through a range of practices and theoretical discussions. They did not emerge at the same time, yet they were mutually reinforcing as descriptive terms of melancholia in the late nineteenth century. The nineteenth-century origins of depression as a mental symptom were considered in Chapter 3. Mental pain has an equally multifaceted history that can be traced in part to early modern religious texts, and in part to physiology, whence it was borrowed as an analogy to describe an emotional state that was perceived as a psychological equivalent of physical pain. The physiological notion of mental pain was more complex, however, as within the new physiological psychology (outlined in Chapter 2), the 'mental' was not merely abstract, but rather understood as the manifestation of physiological processes in the brain. 'Suicidal tendencies', conversely, have more clearly traceable roots, becoming a prominent symptom through the medical certificates of insanity that were introduced in the early decades of the nineteenth century, and through which it became a significant statistical marker for melancholic patients.

A strong link was forged in the mid-to-late nineteenth century between melancholia and mental pain, depression, and suicidality, and, to a lesser extent, religious delusions. This relationship proved useful in a number of ways, two of which are of particular significance for the present story. First, it played a key role in the nosological reification and standardisation of melancholia in late Victorian medico-psychological literature. Secondly, it offered a useful tool within endeavours to establish psychological medicine (later psychiatry) as a modern scientific discipline and branch of medicine. While this story is focussed on the British context, it is important to note that the standardisation of melancholia was not a strictly domestic development. British physicians read the works of many of their European counterparts; journals were increasingly publishing English translations of foreign (chiefly German, French, and Italian) articles, and ideas and concepts from continental psychiatry were appropriated by British medical psychologists to various extents. In much of the literature, mental pain and depression were held up as a driving force in the suicidality of simple, non-delusional melancholia, whereas religious delusions, particularly a belief in having committed 'the unpardonable sin', was perceived as triggering suicidal intent in people suffering from more severe forms of the disease. This chapter traces these themes through some of the most widely read textbooks of mental disease to emerge in late Victorian Britain by influential medical psychologists such as Henry Maudsley and George Savage, as well as through a number of journal case studies on melancholia published in the last few decades of the nineteenth century.

Central to the standardisation of melancholia was the growing use of medical statistics. The practice of collecting and disseminating patient data in numerical tabular form played a key role in the development of diagnostic practices in the mid-to-late nineteenth century. As will be seen below, in the case of melancholia, this is illustrated by the emphasis placed on suicidality as a symptom of the disease, and by the use of simple key terms to describe a patient's mental state, in particular 'depression'. Historians have drawn upon the large body of asylum statistics that emerged in the wake of the creation of the Lunacy Commission in 1845 in attempts to recreate the Victorian asylum milieu and make sense of the practices and experiences of doctors and patients. However, despite the wealth of existing research into the nineteenth-century lunacy trade and the key role asylum statistics has played in such research, the relationship between statistical knowledge and diagnostic theory and practices remains remarkably underexplored. Lunacy administration, statistical collecting and reporting, and the dissemination of clinical data in professional fora such as meetings, journals, and textbooks were key processes in the creation of modern diagnostic categories. Two events in particular facilitated the reification of melancholia as a modern biomedical mental disease with a relatively standardised set of diagnostic criteria. The first of these was the creation of a large body of asylum statistics, as well as increasingly standardised practices for recording symptoms. The second was the emergence of a professional community of medical psychologists, where the question of classification was widely debated, and whence a vast field of published material on nosological and diagnostic questions was emerging. The apparent prevalence of 'suicidal propensities' in patients diagnosed with melancholia serves here as an illustration of the role of administrative practices, chiefly statistical reporting, in the standardisation of melancholia in this period.

Statistics and classification were contentious topics among late Victorian asylum doctors, and lively discussions took place at meetings of the Medico-Psychological Association, as well as on the pages of its periodical, the *Journal of Mental Science*. Such debates occurred at a time when British alienists were trying to assert the status of their profession as a medical science and academic discipline. Yet, while published articles and textbooks flourished, gradually establishing a solid theoretical framework for psychological medicine, debates regarding asylum admission, treatment, diagnosis, and protection of patients tell of a profession where doubts and anxieties were pervasive and answers few. This chapter begins with a look at the emergence and reification of suicidality as a key symptom of melancholia in the second half of the century, and the role played by statistics in this development. It then maps two of the other key symptoms referred to above—mental pain, and religious delusions—asking how these became part of an increasingly standardised definition of melancholia. Finally, the chapter concludes by discussing the increasingly coherent diagnosis that emerged in the last decade of the century, and the growing medical attention brought to bear upon simple or non-delusional melancholia, a mental state that straddled the boundary between normal and pathological emotions.

The next and final chapter follows the narrative presented here to the pages of asylum casebooks, where the key symptoms of melancholia were seen to manifest in a wide range of acts and expressions. Taken together,

the last two chapters of this book aim to highlight a tension within psychiatric classification that has been a feature of this kind of knowledge since
its inception. They show how, on the one hand, the defining symptoms
of melancholia emerged as melancholic patients frequently manifested
behaviour that appeared to indicate that they suffered from pathological low mood, painful emotions, and thoughts of suicide. In this way,
an increasingly standardised symptomatology can be seen as a response
to 'typical' psychological phenomena clustering together in a significant
section of asylum populations. On the other hand, however, the perceived
need for coherent diagnostic categories, swifter recording practices, and
more efficient data collection, created an environment in which a vast
range of human acts and expressions were increasingly interpreted as
homogenous and made to fit the standard description of melancholia
with its key criteria. What these chapters—and the book as a whole—
aim to show, then, is that the emergence of a key set of criteria for
melancholia that centred on low mood and suicidality was not inevitable,
but neither was the diagnosis simply 'constructed'. The production of
knowledge about human beings is always a complex, negotiated, multifaceted process, and the creation of modern mood disorders, of which
nineteenth-century melancholia was the first, is no exception.

THE PROBLEM OF DIAGNOSIS
IN PSYCHOLOGICAL MEDICINE

British textbooks on mental disease greatly proliferated in the last two
decades of the nineteenth century, with a growing number of asylum
physicians deciding to turn their clinical experience into educational material for students and fellow practitioners. It is difficult to speak of the
'standard' psychiatric textbook as physicians differed a great deal in their
approach to mental disease, both in terms of diagnostics and treatment
as well as aetiology and internal explanatory models. Nevertheless, a
few general remarks can be made about the late Victorian textbook of
insanity. First, while aetiology and treatment were undoubtedly significant areas of psychiatric knowledge, far more attention was devoted to
diagnostics, that is, the question of how to identify various forms of
mental disease. It follows that textbooks were overwhelmingly devoted
to classification. Secondly, different asylums deployed different diagnostic
systems, with variations being national, regional, local, and even individual

to each physician. At the same time, a measure of de facto standardisation was gradually instituted, in part as a result of Lunacy Commission recommendations and directives. Textbooks and articles also suggest that a gradual consensus emerged around major diagnostic categories such as melancholia, mania, and general paralysis. Thirdly, the melancholia diagnosis received growing attention in many British textbooks in the last quarter of the century, and diagnostic descriptions became increasingly homogenous, coalescing around mental depression and suicidal tendencies as the core distinguishing symptoms of melancholia. Fourthly, the process of creating and reifying diagnostic categories was complex and contested, depending upon a number of factors: formal guidelines relating to recording practices, statistical tables, growing concern for patient safety and the often conflicting concern for patient liberty, as well as contradictory systems of knowledge (e.g. religious versus scientific, lay versus medical). Equally important, however, were such mundane factors as habit and convenience, made all the more significant with the introduction of standardised printed forms for recording symptoms and diagnoses.

At a time when an increasing number of asylum physicians chose to publish books and articles on their research and clinical experience, nosological concerns were at the forefront of professional debates. What kind of system one adhered to was a statement about one's epistemological approach to insanity—as Maudsley had suggested in 1867, a correct classification system was one that was grounded in scientific knowledge and 'in conformity with nature'.[15] But what 'nature' suggested about the classification of mental disease was not universally self-evident. A rapidly expanding catalogue of publications on insanity meant a rapidly growing number of different systems. From the multitude of nuances and more marked differences between nosologies, three ways of labelling and categorising insanity can be identified that were particularly common: classification according to stages (e.g. acute or chronic), classification according to causes (e.g. alcoholic insanity, puerperal insanity, climacteric insanity), and classification according to observable symptoms (e.g. melancholia, mania, general paralysis). Many physicians used a combination of all three, rather than selecting one, and all three systems prevailed in some form or another throughout the Victorian period. What is perhaps most telling about the different systems proposed is that the one thing physicians largely agreed on was the difficulty in translating clinical observations into consistent theoretical frameworks. To label and cate-gorise the multitude of human activity that was met with on asylum and hospital wards was a challenging task. Henry Monro noted as much in the 1850s:

> All who have charge of asylums must well know how very different the clear and distinct classification of books is from that medley of symptoms which is presented by real cases, where each case seems to bear as peculiarly its own idiosyncrasies of detail, as hardly to allow of very minute division.[16]

Nevertheless, despite their own admission as to the problems inherent in trying to attach strict medical labels to the unpredictability of human emotions and actions, Victorian medical psychologists remained persuaded of the necessity and usefulness of classification, setting the tone for psychiatric diagnosis ever since.

CLASSIFICATION AND MEDICAL STATISTICS

While many British physicians were keen to add their own version of popular nosologies to the ever-growing catalogue of systems, a universal system of classification was proposed in the 1844 report of the Metropolitan Commissioners in Lunacy to the Lord Chancellor. The Metropolitan Commission had been set up in 1828 by the Madhouses Act to oversee the management of lunatic asylums and licensed houses in London and surrounding areas,[17] with its authority extended to all of England and Wales in 1842.[18] The nosology presented in the report brought together old and new categories, suggesting nine different types of mental disease: mania (divided into acute, ordinary, and periodical), dementia, melancholia, monomania, moral insanity, congenital idiocy, congenital imbecility, general paralysis, and epilepsy. The report remarked that melancholia, monomania, and moral insanity were 'sometimes comprehended under the term Partial Insanity', and further suggested that 'delirium tremens' might be considered as an additional category to those stated. Despite numerous individual attempts by physicians to put forward their system of classification as the most 'correct' and 'scientific', a somewhat simplified version of the nosology endorsed by the London Commissioners proved enduring in the context of asylum diagnostics. Its apparent popularity can be explained in large part through the requirements placed on asylum medical officers by the Lunacy Commission in the second half of the century, as will be seen below.

In its 1844 report, the Metropolitan Commission emphasised the importance and value of statistics in the management of asylums. The report lamented the inconsistent nature of existing figures, which were perceived as incomplete and fragmentary, failing to give an accurate account of the number of lunatics residing in Britain. Following from this, an inquiry was undertaken, whereby the managers of asylums and licensed houses in England and Wales were asked to supply their latest figures, with the investigation being extended 'to a certain degree, to Scotland and Ireland'. In order that such inquiries could be carried out more efficiently and comprehensively in the future, the Commissioners proposed the nationwide introduction of 'certain forms of Registers and Medical Books, to be kept at all Asylums, with a view to the preparation of Statistical Returns, at stated and uniform periods'.[19] When the national Lunacy Commission was created in 1845 (see below), such a system was rapidly instituted, and had significant and lasting consequences for how melancholia was defined and diagnosed.

The classification and diagnosis of melancholia took place against the backdrop of a wider context of a culture increasingly preoccupied with categories and numbers.[20] The natural historians of the eighteenth century, such as Linnaeus and Blumenbach, had cemented classification as a central component of their work; to know the living world, one must organise it—name, label, and categorise it. When Linnaeus put together his *Systema Naturae*, he considered his own work to be that of an identifier, whose task it was to find the correct boxes for each thing existing in nature.[21] As Foucault has suggested, however, the birth of modern classification 'was not an age-old inattentiveness being suddenly dissipated, but a new field of visibility being constituted in all its density'.[22] In the nineteenth century classification became a totalising practice; '[p]eople classified, measured, and standardized just about everything – animals, human races, books, pharmaceutical products, taxes, jobs, and diseases'.[23]

Classification of mental disease was helped by another nineteenth-century favourite preoccupation: statistics.[24] Terrence Murphy has traced the early years of modern statistics among French scientists such as Condorcet, who hoped to establish 'a science of decision making', a tool with which decisions in political society could be made according to calculated probability and thus protected from rash judgments motivated by passion.[25] Numbers would tell people which course of sociopolitical action to take by suggesting probable consequences of various options. While Condorcet did not complete his visionary project of a decision-making science, the foundation was laid, and others continued to build upon it, most notably Laplace.[26]

The theory of probability was picked up and utilised by Philippe Pinel, who had taken over the running of Paris' large asylums during the first republic. Pinel believed that persistent recording of data that allowed the medical scientist to compare and contrast symptoms and their treatments would result in improved therapeutics and consequently better outcomes for those diagnosed with various forms of insanity. He separated medicine into two branches, nosography and therapeutics, suggesting that proba-bility theory applied only to the latter.[27] Some decades later, however, it became productive of the former. In the second half of the century, reasoning about the regularity of events became paramount to the diag-nosis of melancholia, and in particular to the almost universal belief that suicidality was a defining symptom of the disease. According to statistics produced by British asylums, expressions and actions collated under the term 'suicidal tendencies' were seen to occur in the disease with frequent regularity, resulting in the expectation that a diagnosis of melancholia meant the likely presence of suicidality. This assumption significantly affected how such patients were cared for—if melancholic patients were expected to harbour suicidal intentions, strict precautions must be taken to ensure that they were unable to injure themselves. It also altered the interpretation of symptoms at the moment of diagnosis. 'Suicidal tenden-cies' became central to the ontology of melancholia—but this was not a simple or inevitable development. It relied upon, and was produced by, a set of legal guidelines generating changes to recording practices and vast amounts of new kinds of statistical data.

ASYLUM STATISTICS AND THE STANDARDISATION OF RECORDING PRACTICES

Wynn's Act of 1808 had allowed for county asylums to be established as institutions providing for pauper lunatics.[28] In the subsequent years, admission to licensed private houses came to require legal documenta-tion certifying the mental state of the person taken into care, a provision that was eventually extended to pauper asylums.[29] As noted above, insti-tutions in the Greater London area had since the late 1820s been subject to inspections and directives from the Metropolitan Commission, which had its powers extended to oversee the running of asylums throughout England and Wales in the last two years of its existence. When the Lunatics Care and Treatment Act and Regulation of Asylums Act[30] (hereafter 'the Lunacy Acts') were passed in 1845, these constituted to a degree 'a consolidation of "lunacy reform"' begun at the end of the previous century.[31] Such earlier developments can also be seen as the first bricks in the bureaucracy that was rapidly constructed in the aftermath of the Acts. Every county in England and Wales was compelled to erect its own pauper asylum within three years. The Acts moreover created a permanent body, the Lunacy Commission, to oversee the implementation of the Acts.[32] While the practice of collecting and disseminating statistical information pertaining to asylum populations had begun under the administration of the Metropolitan Commissioners, with the creation of its successor body this process became vastly more comprehensive, organised, systematised, detailed, regular, and wide-reaching. In the first instance, the yearly reports that asylums were required to submit to the Commission produced a wealth of statistical information about the people residing in these institutions. In addition to this, almost immediately after the initial stipulations of the Acts had come into force these were built upon through a relentless flow of circular letters from the Commission to the asylums requesting various kinds of information, from 'a copy of your present Diet Table'[33] to whether post-mortem examinations were performed on a regular basis.[34]

The Lunacy Acts had set out detailed instructions for the management of asylum populations, including the various administrative tasks required, and attached to the main documents were a number of appendices with templates for some of the paperwork relating to admission and care of lunatics under the new law. Of primary concern for the present story are the medical certificates of insanity and accompanying reception orders, as well as the asylum admissions registers and casebooks. The 1845 Lunacy Acts extended the scope of medical certificates and explicitly set out their legal framework. The Acts stipulated that a patient admitted to the asylum must be legally certified as 'a lunatic [or an insane person, or an idiot, or a person of unsound mind] and a proper person to be confined'.[35] They distinguished between private and pauper patients; for the latter one certificate was enough, while for the former two (signed by different physicians) were required.[36] Appendices to the Acts provided doctors with a clear template for the medical certificate and reception order, the latter listing the various 'particulars' required, such as 'age', 'sex', 'place of abode', whether this was the patient's 'first attack', and whether he or she was 'epileptic', 'suicidal', or 'dangerous to others'.[37] In the case of private patients, this statement was often filled out by a spouse, relative, or friend, while reception orders belonging to pauper patients were customarily filled out and signed by a magistrate or workhouse official. Upon arrival at the asylum, the data on these forms would be transferred to the admissions register. Asylum physicians were legally required to add a diagnosis to this information within a week of admission.[38]

Following the establishment of the Lunacy Commission, asylum physicians were obliged to compile yearly reports on the state of their institutions, including statistics on a large number of aspects pertaining to the asylum population. This meant that for the first time a large body of data was created from which one could extract virtually any thinkable piece of information about every county asylum in Britain,[39] organised in tabular numerical form. Asylum physicians, the county Board of Visitors,[40] and Lunacy Commissioners were able to learn from such figures how many men and women resided in each asylum, what proportion of these were married, single, or widowed, which professions and religious persuasions were represented among them, the average age of patients, the most common form of mental disease (usually mania), how many people were admitted and discharged each year, how many patients died in the asylum and how many autopsies were performed, what treatments were administered, and so on.

One of the provisions set out in the Lunacy Care and Treatments Act of 1845 was that each asylum had to keep a casebook where detailed information about each patient's condition was to be entered at regular intervals. The instructions of the Act had been relatively vague regarding the casebook, stating merely that such a book should be kept by every asylum and that the presiding physician should in this book 'from time to time make entries of the mental state and bodily condition of each patient, together with a correct description of the medicine and other remedies prescribed for his disorder'.[41] Shortly after the Lunacy Acts had come into force, however, the secretary of the Commission sent out a letter to all county asylums with guidelines on the use of the casebook, which were subsequently also incorporated into an 1853 legal amendment. The Commissioners left the format of the casebook to be decided by each superintendent, since a strict template 'might tend to cramp and fetter the Practitioner in his detail of individual cases'. However, clear directives were provided concerning the content of the casebook. Physicians were instructed to enter much of the basic information derived from the admissions register, such as name, sex, and occupation of the patient. Secondly, a detailed description of the patient's external bodily condition, and of respiratory and visceral organs, was to be given, along with a pulse and state of the tongue and skin. Thirdly,

> A description of the phenomena of mental disorder which characterize the case; – the manner and period of the attack; – with a minute account of the symptoms, and the changes produced in the patient's temper or disposition; – specifying whether the malady displays itself by any, and what, illusions, or by irrational conduct, or morbid and dangerous habits and propensities'.[42]

Bearing in mind, then, that the Lunacy Acts had already stipulated that for each patient a diagnosis had to be entered; this diagnosis also had to be accompanied by a detailed description of the disease, listing emotional and intellectual symptoms, as well as noting whether the patient was considered to harbour any 'morbid propensities'.

With the Lunacy Commission's strong emphasis on the importance of collecting and disseminating statistics, asylum physicians inevitably devoted a considerable amount of time and energy to the gathering of such data, and consequently also to discussions about how to best go about this task. Statistics became a central topic of discussion at the annual meetings of the Medico-Psychological Association. Unlike in Germany, where a number of different psychiatric associations and journals had been created at this time (sometimes in opposition to each other),[43] the Medico-Psychological Association was the chief forum within which British asylum physicians could meet and discuss their trade and their nascent discipline. Its professional periodical, the *Journal of Mental Science*, offered a space for physicians working in the field of psychological medicine to present their research and partake of and comment on the work of others. The *Journal of Mental Science* moreover published the proceedings from the Association's quarterly and annual meetings.

In 1864, the members of the Association appointed a committee consisting of Henry Maudsley, C. Lockhart Robertson (of the Sussex County Asylum at Hayward's Heath), and John Thurnam (of Wiltshire County Asylum) whose task it was to look into the question of data collection in the asylum, and consequently 'to draw up a series of tables, and a form of register which might be the basis of a uniform system of asylum statistics'. The intention was that 'these tables be submitted to the Commissioners' who would be 'asked to sanction and promulgate them'. The Committee of Asylum Statistics proposed six tables, revised from those already in use and intended to homogenise and streamline asylum statistics. The tables concerned statistics on admissions, discharges, and deaths, but did not include columns for specific diagnoses.[44] At the Association's annual meeting in 1867, the Committee was pleased to report that twenty-six English asylums, two Scottish, and one Irish had adopted the new tables.[45] These had also received the blessing of the Commissioners in Lunacy, who praised the initiative of the Medico-Psychological Association in facilitating the collection of numerical data from asylums around the country, and who had endorsed the new tables in their annual report the previous year.[46] The Commissioners suggested that in addition to the existing tables, it would also be 'desirable' to draw up uniform tables showing 'the ages of patients on admission, the duration of the exiting attack, and the form of mental disorder under which they labour', expressing 'hope' that 'the medical officers of asylums may see the great importance of coming to some agreement upon these points'.[47]

The Committee on Asylum statistics proposed three additional tables that partially redressed the Lunacy Commission's concerns. New forms asked for causes of insanity to be listed, as well as length and number of attacks, and causes of death. The latter included indications of the type of disorder that the deceased patient had suffered from with the heading 'maniacal or melancholic exhaustion or decay' listed alongside other causes such as 'epilepsy', 'apoplexy', and 'general paresis'.[48] However, the Medico-Psychological Association failed to adopt a uniform system of classification of mental disease; not surprisingly, perhaps, considering the vastly conflicting and diverse opinions of its members on this matter. In the 1879 edition of his textbook, Henry Maudsley remarked that 'as many as forty or fifty different systems of classification have been propounded',[49] and the problems attached to developing a correct system were, he suggested, the same as in the 1840s and 50s: 'until we know exactly the obscure constitutional conditions which are at the bottom of the differences of symptoms – of which we know nothing yet – we cannot dispense with a symptomatological classification'.[50] George Savage echoed this claim a few years later, adding that he himself chose to use the system that was most 'convenient' from a clinical point of view.[51]

The problem of uniform classification was not in the end to be resolved through theoretical discussions in the forum of the Medico-Psychological Association or in textbooks or journal articles. Rather, the instituting of practices aimed at facilitating the collection and coherence of medical statistics had the effect of producing a de facto standardised nosology. While physicians themselves were unable or unwilling to agree on a nationwide system of classification, the increasing number of directives issued from the Lunacy Commission regarding the collection of asylum statistics encouraged the use of certain specified categories. In the 1870s the Lunacy Commission introduced pre-printed forms for recording the different types of mental disease in the asylum. As noted above, medical officers were already required by law to record a diagnosis in the casebook within one week of a patient's admission, and this information was included in each asylum's annual report to the Commission. However, with different nosologies favoured by different physicians, cross-comparison between asylums in this area was blatantly problematic. In an attempt to redress this, attached to a circular letter sent out to all asylums and licensed houses in 1876 was a pre-printed form for the main register of patients, with five columns provided under the heading 'form of mental disorder': mania, melancholia, dementia, congenital insanity, and 'other forms of insanity' (general paralysis was also listed, but as a symptom alongside epilepsy rather than as a separate disease entity).[52]

While the implementation of directives from the Commission necessarily varied between asylums, and while some physicians were more likely to make frequent use of the last column than others, the Commissioners' persistent attempts to derive uniform, comparable data from asylums were crucial in shaping what kind of data was recorded. Melancholia was a term that had existed in medical literature in some form or another since antiquity, it was recognisable and came, increasingly, with a number of well-known features attached to it. The two most easily distinguishable types of insanity on the asylum wards were generally considered to be melancholia and mania. That the Commission's pre-printed table listed these two categories was significant in ensuring their continued usage on the wards. Consequently, a sample survey of statistics from a number of asylums around the country between the 1860s and 1880s indicate that the two most common forms of mental disease diagnosed were mania and melancholia (in that order).[53] While physicians continued to battle out their disagreements over classification in journal articles and at professional gatherings, it can nonetheless be concluded that by the 1870s the beginnings of a standard nosology existed in Britain, one which held melancholia to be a distinct form of mental disease. Mid-to-late Victorian physicians offered concise diagnostic descriptions of melancholia which, in contrast to those of earlier writers like Conolly, centred upon the definition of a disease entity, rather than of the person(s) seen to embody the illness. Despite persisting disagreements over what kind of system should be used, the nosological status of melancholia was conversely strengthened and homogenised during this period.

MELANCHOLIA AND SUICIDAL TENDENCIES

While physicians might have preferred to use their own system of classification, they were nevertheless keen on using the statistical data collected for their annual reports to the Commission in their own theoretical discussions on mental pathology. Such information overwhelmingly suggested that a majority of melancholic patients harboured suicidal tendencies, and of all patients admitted to the asylum, the majority of those who received the 'suicidal' label were diagnosed with melancholia. In the first half of the century physicians across Europe had become increasingly preoccupied with suicide and insanity, as illustrated by Forbes Winslow's popular *The Anatomy of Suicide* published in 1840. Winslow's work was a comprehensive lesson in suicide statistics, making the most of the science of numbers as a tool for explaining why people would commit what had long been an unforgivable sin but which was now more frequently perceived as the product of an unsound mind. Winslow, Esquirol, Falret, and other early nineteenth-century medical scientists with an interest in suicide had two things in common. First, they were almost exclusively concerned with completed suicides, and the statistics they compiled and/or drew upon were of people who had died (presumably) at their own hands. The adjective 'suicidal' was a recent addition to the English language. It was used sparingly in the first few decades of the century, but by the late 1800s it had become a standard diagnostic term. Secondly, they paid only marginal attention to suicide in relation to melancholia.

This was in stark contrast to their late nineteenth-century successors. In the last two decades of the nineteenth century, 'suicidal tendencies' became a defining symptom of melancholia.[54] This shift can in part be attributed to one of the obligatory questions on the reception order which accompanied the medical certificates of insanity. As noted above, the reception order required a yes or no answer as to whether the patient to be admitted was 'suicidal'. Once the suicidal label had been affixed to the individual certified as a lunatic, it followed them into the asylum casebook, where it was noted together with other symptoms, bodily condition, and diagnosis. This information became part of each asylum's annual statistical reports, which indicated that a significant portion of patients were considered suicidal. This category of patients became a particular concern of the Commissioners in Lunacy; suicidal patients posed a threat to the reputation of each asylum and thus to the competency of the Commission.

Less than a decade after the passing of the Lunacy Acts, Thomas Brushfield, medical superintendent at Parkside Cheshire County asylum (and later at Brookwood in Surrey), concluded from his annual data that 42 out of the 102 patients admitted to Parkside that year were recorded as having exhibited 'suicidal impulses'.[55] Alluding to the significance such figures were rapidly taking on for physicians and Commissioners alike, he suggested that '[t]his class at all times causes great anxiety to the medical officers, as notwithstanding the greatest vigilance on the part of the attendants, fatal cases will sometimes occur; no instance of the kind has, however, happened during the past year'.[56] Parkside was representative of the norm. The figures reported to the Lunacy Commission and the Scottish Board of Commissioners from British asylums each year showed a persistently high (and rising) level of 'suicidal propensities' in patients diagnosed with melancholia.

Anxieties generated by asylum statistics led to an increasing focus on prevention. Patients considered to harbour suicidal tendencies were assigned a pink caution card to be worn at all times, and extra night duty staff were deployed to ensure that suicidal patients were never left unsupervised.[57] Concerns about how to best care for suicidal patients also led to a revival in support for mechanical restraint, a practice that had been rejected by the new 'humanitarian' practice of moral treatment that had emerged at the turn of the nineteenth century. As the relationship between melancholia and suicidality gradually became circular and mutually constitutive, the necessity of restraining such patients for their own good was increasingly presented as a key argument for having melancholy and suicidal patients admitted to the asylum. Physicians were expected to treat patients and keep them safe, meaning that a suicide within the walls of an asylum, or resulting from an escape, was a black stain on that institution's reputation. At the same time, however, there was political opposition to restraint, as well as to arbitrary confinement. Tension also existed between the workhouse and the asylum, with disagreement over who should ultimately be responsible for the treatment of pauper lunatics. The relationship between these two institutions had consequences for the emergence of suicidality as a medical concept and defining symptom of melancholia. For a troublesome patient to be transferred from the (usually more crowded and comparatively scarcely resourced) workhouse infirmary to the asylum, the staff at the former generally had to be able to demonstrate that the patient could not be properly cared for or managed in the workhouse. This was most easily done by affirming that the patient was a danger to other residents, or to themselves—in other words, 'suicidal'.

Concerns about a patient's suicidal intent were not, however, alleviated by their presence in the asylum. The Commissioners in Lunacy, whose responsibility it was to ensure that Britain's lunatics were properly cared for, were anxious about potential suicides in the asylum, and consequently instructed medical officers to ensure that such patients were being appropriately watched over. Death by suicide was, in fact, rare in the asylum; nevertheless, preoccupation with statistics over suicidal tendencies grew steadily in the decades following the 1845 Acts. The Commissioners took measures to ensure that concern over and precautions against suicidality were a priority in every asylum by repeatedly emphasising the matter in their correspondence with asylum medical officers.[58]

There was, however, some controversy surrounding the suicidal label, particularly in regard to the reliability of asylum data on the prevalence of suicidality. Bethlem superintendent George Savage questioned the justification to keep suicidal patients under constant surveillance on the basis that the statistics on suicidality were flawed. Many patients who were given the suicidal label upon certification or admission were not, he argued, 'actively suicidal'. While 'many speak of suicide', he said, 'but few really determine to attempt it'.[59] Consequently, he concluded that 'I do not think that more than five per cent of our admissions are "actively suicidal"'.[60] Many of his peers were equally critical of the validity of statistics. While the members of the Medico-Psychological Association had made efforts to comply with the Lunacy Commission's requirements for the recording and collecting of statistical data, many physicians expressed scepticism about the usefulness of such numerical information. At the 1865 annual meeting of the Association, a number of its members became involved in a discussion about the 'fallaciousness' of statistics, which led Henry Monro to declare that 'of all the humbugs of the present day

that of statistics is the greatest'.[61] Most of the members who partici-
pated in the discussion were in agreement that figures collected were too
diverse, fragmented, and arbitrary for any meaningful cross-comparison
to be made between asylums. Maudsley summed up what appeared to be
the general sentiment of the group when he ventured that numerical data
was 'generally so insufficient as to be not only not useful but positively to
mislead. Strictly comparable cases are not taken; conditions and circumstances of importance are neglected, or are not observed as they should
be, so that the statistics lose all their value, and are positively used for the
purpose of inculcating what is not true'. While he suggested that statistics could indeed be useful 'if properly collected', he implored his peers to
remember that they 'never do establish laws or exact facts of any kind'.[62]
The sciences of classification and statistics were undoubtedly embraced
by nineteenth-century medical psychologists, but it would be wrong to
assume that the adoption of these practices occurred in an uncontested
and unproblematic way. On the contrary, the role and the reliability of
statistics in the diagnosis and treatment of mental disease was a topic of
contention among Victorian physicians.

Brushfield, who had moved to Brookwood asylum in Surrey in 1869,
echoed Maudsley's warning in one of his annual reports to the Lunacy
Commission. He suggested that the flawed nature of statistics on suicidal
patients were due to the way this data was collected.[63] As noted above,
the reception order accompanying the medical certificates of insanity
required an answer to the question of whether the person to be certified was 'epileptic, suicidal or dangerous to others'. Unlike the 'facts
indicating insanity' on the medical certificate, which was filled out by a
physician, the information requested on the reception order was usually
provided by a relative, friend, or workhouse official. Moreover, the
format of the two documents differed significantly. If reliable data was
to be collected, he argued, these discrepancies had to be addressed.[64]
In their present state, the forms resulted in incorrect information about
a patient's mental state, in particular relating to suicidality, as the forms
obscured a distinction between patients who were 'a danger to themselves', conflating the patients with 'no suicidal motive' who nonetheless
'imperils his own life by various acts', and those with genuine 'suicidal
tendencies'. He illustrated the first category with the case of a woman
who was admitted to the asylum after having 'cut her left hand off because
she thought it was Scripturally wrong'. While this patient was described

as 'suicidal' on her certificate, the label was incorrect since her motive for mutilating herself was 'a non-suicidal one'.[65]

When it came to suicidal melancholics, however, Brushfield was clear, declaring that 'I would urge upon all medical practitioners the necessity of regarding all cases of melancholia as having suicidal tendencies'. Such tendencies could be deduced from patient interviews as well as from conversations with friends and relatives, and these should, he argued, be cited on the medical certificate under the section requesting the 'facts indicating insanity'.[66] He went on to suggest what such facts might consist of Suicidal tendencies in melancholic patients could manifest, he argued, in the expression of 'melancholy views', especially of a religious nature, such as believing oneself to have committed sins, or more overtly in the form of attempts at self-destruction.[67]

The question on the reception order requiring a yes or no answer to whether the lunatic was suicidal merged a wide range of acts and behaviours into this category. This homogenising process was at the same time productive of a wealth of purported psychopathological knowledge about the people to whom these categories were seen to apply. As will be seen in Chapter 6, a vast number of acts and expressions were collapsed into the single term 'suicidal', such as talking about death, refusal of food, thoughts of guilt and damnation, fear of persecution, and self-inflicted bodily harm. Increasingly exact knowledge was produced by allowing standardised categories to obscure the eclectic nature of human life that terms like 'suicidal' were deployed to explain. By mapping the work done by standardised forms and recording practices we can learn something about the process whereby 'a seemingly neutral data collection mechanism is substituted for ethical conflict about the contents of the forms'. When this occurs, then, 'the moral debate is partially erased. One may get ever more precise knowledge, without having resolved deeper questions, and indeed, by burying those questions'.[68] Through the recording practices and data collection in asylums following the creation of the new bureaucracy presided over by the Lunacy Commission the term 'suicidal' simplified and obscured the complex and varied; it neutralised the contested and conflicted.

When statistical data from reception orders and medical certificates was merged with information derived from asylum case notes and registers, this showed that the 'suicidal' label was applied more frequently to people diagnosed with melancholia than to any other disease category. This facilitated the argument that melancholics were by far the most suicidal of all lunatics. Eventually this argument became self-perpetuating, and physicians began to suspect suicidal tendencies in melancholic patients even when these were not openly manifested. In this way, suicidality went from being a marginal symptom of melancholia early in the century, to becoming a key defining criteria of the condition on par with 'depression'. Suicidality and melancholia became mutually constitutive: increasingly the presence of one was enough for the 'discovery' of the other.

THE HISTORICAL ROOTS OF 'MENTAL PAIN'

While the emergence of suicidality as a defining symptom of melancholia was closely tied to the medical certificates of insanity and the growing body of asylum statistics, 'mental pain' had rather different origins. Mental pain was conceived of as analogous to somatic pain, and like the latter had a solid biomedical explanation and trajectory. However, the patients to whom the melancholia diagnosis was affixed appeared to speak of their pain as something quite different. Patients' own expressions of sin and guilt, and stories offered by distressed relatives and spouses, were interpreted by physicians and presented in medical language. This practice of interspersing curt keyword descriptions of symptoms with verbatim patient quotations created a language of diagnosis and classification in which medical and lay descriptions were awkwardly fused. This is equally apparent in descriptions of religious delusions as a symptom of melancholia, as will be seen below. Both mental pain and religious delusions as symptoms of melancholia illustrate the tension between spiritual and scientific worldviews in the period, reflecting a culture where the two were simultaneously conflicting and closely intertwined.[69] In the late nineteenth century the term mental pain was deployed by physicians as a predominantly biological description of melancholic suffering, but its meaning had gradually shifted from earlier spiritual language to eventually enter medico-scientific nomenclature through early modern medical writings that more comfortably straddled the emerging divide between scientific and spiritual conceptions of the human condition.

Much existing scholarly work on the history of pain is concerned with the medieval and early modern periods[70]; however, a rich literature has begun to emerge that seeks to historicise nineteenth- and twentieth-century conceptions of pain.[71] Javier Moscoso's *Pain: A Cultural History* (2012) addresses ontological evolutions of pain from medieval Christian conceptions to modern scientific ones. With the advent of nineteenth-century scientific medicine, he perceives a shift whereby the sufferer's 'private experience' was objectified through new ways of constituting, explaining, and labelling pain. In a context where pain, like so many other aspects of society, had to be measurable, there was no room for 'unjustified claims and disproportionate laments' from the suffering subject. 'As opposed to introspection and testimony', he argues, 'the new science of the intimate sense had to be rooted in physiology and physics'.[72] What emerged within psychological medicine, however, was a more complex picture. The circular relationship between clinical practice and theoretical discussions created a space within which psychological pain was constituted as physiological, and as an object that could be recorded and measured in statistical tables. Yet doctors were only able to access the nature of this mental pain through patient testimony. The trouble of recording and diagnosing the abstract pain of emotional life lay in the fact that its chief manifestation was through language, which revealed nothing about the internal neural processes that were believed to be the 'real' source of patients' mental pain.

An important consequence of medico-psychological perceptions of the mental suffering that melancholic patients expressed as one having traceable (but regrettably not observable) physiological roots, was that any references to God, sin, and divine retribution were translated into patient journals and medical literature as 'religious delusions'. However, when mapping the shifting meanings of mental pain from earlier non-medical usages to its later emergence as physiological metaphor and finally a psychological phenomenon with an explicable biological basis, the source of the melancholic patient's perception becomes apparent. In a series of letters written at the turn of the eighteenth century, clergyman and religious thinker John Norris and philosopher Mary Astell[73] debated the relationship between mental pain and sin. Astell asserted that 'I cannot form to my self any Idea of Sin which does not include in it the greatest Pain and Misery'. Committing a sin against God would, she argued, result in mental pain. In much the same way as 'a musical Instrument, if it were capable of Sense and Thought, would be uneasie and in pain when harsh discordant Notes are play'd upon it; so Man, when he breaks the Law of his Nature, and runs counter to those Motions his Maker has assign'd him...must needs be in Pain and Misery'.[74] For Astell, then, to act against God and nature was to act sinfully and to cause pain. A similar understanding of mental pain as sin was expressed a few years later by another English clergyman, Richard Fiddes, who in his *Fifty Two Practical Discourses on Several Subjects* (1720) explained that 'what I principally here intend, by mental Pain, is, that Anguish and Remorse of Mind, which Sinners so naturally feel, and all of them, more or less, when they call their own Ways to remembrance, and reflect upon their sins.'[75]

It is significant to note the unambiguous way in which this point of view established a causal trajectory between unnatural and ungodly conduct and the experience of mental pain. A century and a half later, British physicians turned this argument on its head, suggesting that the mental pain felt by melancholics would render the act of suicide—the ultimate crime against God and nature—both 'logical' and 'natural'. Victorian medical psychologists were keen to assert the irrelevance of moral judgement when explaining the symptoms and causes of mental disease, but their case notes allude to people for whom the moral implications of their painful emotions were a great source of distress. The association between religion and mental pain was rooted in a centuries-old spiritual worldview where Man's duties to God were foremost, and where to act against divine law was for faithful Christians an unequivocal source of pain and despair. It is not surprising that a relationship between religious morality and emotional distress that had endured in some form or another for centuries appeared to prevail among melancholic patients against medico-scientific explanations that were, by comparison, embryonic.

The medico-psychological understanding of mental pain that emerged in the nineteenth century arose chiefly from a different epistemological context, that of experimental physiology, yet the two conceptions remained in a close and often antagonistic relationship throughout the period. It should also be noted that in early modern literature, spiritual and medical conceptions of pain were not mutually exclusive, and such perceptions were not simply erased with the advent of physiological psychology in the nineteenth century. It follows that early modern ideas about mental pain as an 'evil' or as 'sin' cannot be simply excluded from late nineteenth-century meanings of the term.[76] Moreover, the adoption of mental pain as a medical phenomenon was not a straightforward production of nineteenth-century physiological psychology, but, like the creation of modern physiology itself, a gradual process where old and new terminology was fused to espouse medical theories about body and mind set in current explanatory frameworks.[77]

When mental pain entered the realm of nineteenth-century physiological psychology and psychological medicine, then, it did so from an eclectic past. Victorian medical scientists used the term in specific ways to explain the psychological suffering that was the manifestation of cerebral irritation producing a state of disordered emotion. Earlier chapters showed how the perceived 'irritation' of the cerebral nerves would over time affect the 'tone' of the brain, causing painful emotional and ideational associations to occur. Andrew Hodgkiss has traced the history of 'pain without lesion' in nineteenth-century European medicine, investigating precisely this conception of how mental pain was perceived to materialise. He pays particular attention to how ideas about cerebral irritation and reflexive action functioned to constitute a physiological model for pain without traceable organic cause in the work of Johannes Müller, Wilhelm Griesinger, and Thomas Laycock. Key to making sense of nineteenth-century psycho-physiological conceptions of pain without lesion is, Hodgkiss argues, the argument, proposed by Laycock, that mental sensations alone were enough to cause irritation of the nerves.[78]

Central to psycho-physiological ideas about mental pain favoured by British medical psychologists in the late nineteenth century was a belief that such pain functioned in much the same way as physical pain. In a similar manner to cerebral irritation and psychological reflex action, mental pain in nineteenth-century physiological psychology held the ambiguous status of being at once metaphorical and literal. Experimental data concerned observable bodily reactions, and knowledge derived from empirical research was extrapolated and analogously applied to speak about mental operations—that which could *not* be observed. At the same time, however, analogies were believed to represent what was actually occurring in the brains of people. Terms like 'irritation', 'reflexion', 'tone', and 'pain' when applied to speak of the mind were seen as explicating cerebral processes as well as psychological operations. This can be seen in Griesinger's discussion of mental pain in the second, extended edition of his textbook.[79] He suggested that it resulted from mental irritation, both of the kind that manifested in psychological exaltation, and of its opposite, depression, and that such pain could be triggered by external as well as internal factors. Citing recent experiments by German physiologist Moritz Schiff,[80] Griesinger held that the sensation of pain 'could only be transmitted through the grey substance', suggesting that pain originated in the brain. This explained, he argued, how mental pain could arise endogenously, through a 'special irritation' of the cerebral tissue.[81]

Older meanings did not simply vanish, however, and they continued to facilitate conceptions of self for the melancholic patients to whom this label was affixed. As will be seen below, where patients communicated a spiritual suffering, their physicians saw a physiologically constituted pain that manifested as a psychological phenomenon. Nevertheless, mental pain was a useful medical concept in the building of a solid biomedical foundation for mental disease. The sensation of pain was an important tool in physiological experiments on nervous function, particularly in its relationship with automated muscular reactivity. It was helpful if one could show that the same connection existed between psychological pain and involuntary action. Such arguments became problematic towards the end of the century, however, when physicians focussed their attention on the perceived prominence of suicidal actions in non-delusional melancholics, as will be seen below. It was more difficult to maintain that suicide, suicidal attempts, and suicidal tendencies were morbid impulses (as was often the case earlier in the century) when the subject was believed to be capable of rational thought. In this context, then, suicidality was reconceptualised, so that mental pain and depression came to function as 'logical' and 'rational' causes of suicidal intent in people perceived to suffer from simple (non-delusional) melancholia.

'Religious Delusions' and 'The Unpardonable Sin'

While 'religious delusions' was not put forward as a defining characteristic of melancholia to the same extent as depression, suicidality, and mental pain, this symptom nevertheless featured frequently in published case studies and descriptions of the disorder. Much like the other key symptoms of melancholia, religious delusions became a standardised term that physicians could use in their work that would make sense to their peers and students. These symptom descriptions recorded by physicians in asylum casebooks and drawn from their interpretations of what patients communicated reveal much about the tensions between lay and medical conceptions of self, and about the negotiations that took place when medical scientists attempted to label and categorise their patients' disordered emotionality. Only the medico-psychological expert could correctly interpret this chaos of human experience; it followed that patients' perceptions of their own misery were, for the most part, wrong. Thomas Clouston remarked that:

In nine cases out of ten, melancholic patients assign as a cause of their misery what is not its cause at all. Here it is where their insane delusions, their false ungrounded beliefs, come in. I have analysed the "causes" assigned by melancholics that I have had under my care during the past seven years for their own depression, and I find them to be wrong in ninety per cent of the cases.[82]

This is illustrated by the frequent use of 'religious delusions' as a descriptive term. A large number of patients expressed sin and the wrath of God as the source of their mental suffering. For melancholic patients, these experiences were very real, but for physicians such spiritual explanations were a clear example of patients assigning an incorrect cause to their suffering.

In a case presented by Maudsley in *The Pathology of Mind* as the first of several 'ordinary illustrations of melancholia', a thirty-six-year-old man described as 'religious and of exemplary character' became, according to Maudsley, weighed down by a 'great depression' that soon produced 'blasphemous ideas' in his mind. Despite his best efforts to rid himself of these thoughts they continued to torture him; 'he was much distressed by this state of things, his gloom increased more and more, and at last he concluded that "he had done it," – namely, committed the unpardonable sin'.[83] A belief in having committed 'the unpardonable sin' was repeatedly cited by Victorian physicians as a cause of their patients' suffering, and frequently constituted the focal point of the latter's 'delusions'. The specific nature of this sin was, however, rarely addressed directly; its meaning was firmly rooted in the Christian culture shared by patients and doctors, and appeared to require little explanation. However, while the concept was awarded scant attention in medical literature beyond its repeated appearance as psychological illusion that was a symptom of disease, it was widely discussed by theological writers of the period, both within the Church of England and among the evangelical denominations in Britain and North America.[84]

While 'the unpardonable sin' was a familiar concept in mid-nineteenth-century writings on Christian morality, there appeared to be no clear agreement on exactly what kind of act constituted such a sin, which was often referred to in imprecise terms as a 'sin against the Holy Ghost'. In the first volume of *Sermons*, an 1864 monograph on Christian doctrine, the famous American clergyman and public speaker Henry Ward Beecher sought to settle this matter by providing a clear explanation of what was meant by this notion, suggesting that 'we are to regard the unpardonable sin, not as any one single offence, but as the state of heart which gives rise to conduct that is not pardonable. It is not an action; it is a condition of disposition or heart from which certain kinds of actions are developed'. Beecher's definition illustrates how Victorian melancholics expressed their religious distress, according to how this was interpreted and noted by their physicians. 'The unpardonable sin' appeared to convey a profound sense of guilt, sometimes for an abominable act that the patient claimed to have committed and sometimes for thinking of committing such an act. The overlap between lay and medical conceptions is evident also in Beecher's work—he suggested that an erroneous belief in having committed the unpardonable sin 'sometimes leads to insanity, and often is the leading feature of religious mania'.[85]

George Savage remarked upon the frequency of religious delusions, noting in melancholics 'a strong tendency to explain their misery by means of some text or religious dogma'.[86] However, there existed a particular category of melancholic lunatics, Savage suggested, usually people who had been subject to a severe religious upbringing, particularly in 'narrow religious sects', whom he liked to refer to as 'the unpardonable sinners' in reference to the common delusion discussed above. His idea of what this most abominable of all sins was meant to refer to was notably different from the kinds of explanations offered by Christian thinkers. A man of science, Savage had no qualms about discussing particular sinful acts, and offered a more specific definition of 'the unpardonable sin' than that of 'the state of heart which gives rise to conduct that is not pardonable' given by Beecher. 'In many cases', Savage suggested to his readers, 'it refers to some sexual abuse'. Thus, the idea often arose following a period of excessive masturbation.[87]

While 'the unpardonable sin' was frequently noted by contemporaneous writers as a recurring delusion in melancholia, Savage appeared to be alone in his reference to immoral sexual conduct. Maudsley did, however, elaborate on the historical origins of this delusion, suggesting that the 'conviction of having committed the unpardonable sin' had existed as 'a common delusion of melancholics since the disciples of Christ introduced that doctrine to mankind'. Thus, the same delusion would not have been possible for 'an ancient Greek who was suffering from the same form of disease'; rather, he would have believed himself 'to be pursued by the Furies'.[88] George Blandford, who spent most of his career

in private practices in London, found the presence of this particular delusion to be a useful diagnostic guiding tool, since it suggested 'that the
patient's condition is one of melancholia'.[89] Blandford did not, however,
hold the delusional belief in having committed the unpardonable sin to
be a particular cause of suicidal intent in melancholic patients. Rather,
he suggested that the suicidal tendency was often strongest in patients
suffering from simple, or non-delusional melancholia, but that, on the
whole, all melancholic patients were 'to be looked upon as suicidal'.[90]
As we shall see below, while delusions of guilt were often seen in late
Victorian medico-psychological literature as a driving force in the suicidal
intent of many melancholics, the symptom was equally perceived as being
particularly prominent in individuals suffering from 'simple' melancholia,
where no delusions were present, and in such cases it was the very absence
of delusions that was given as the chief cause of the suicidal tendency.

Nosological Shifts: Maudsley Revisited

Henry Maudsley's published work on mental disease serves as a useful
reference point for the changing character of melancholia in the second
half of the nineteenth century, as it exemplifies many of the wider debates
and tensions that existed in relation to the status and definition of this
diagnosis. When the first edition of Maudsley's textbook on mental physiology and pathology was published in the late 1860s, melancholia was
variably seen as an independent disease category, or as a form of monomania, moral or partial insanity, or as variation of mania proper. As
shown in Chapter 4, in 1867 Maudsley had classified non-delusional
melancholia together with non-delusional mania under 'affective insanity',
while melancholia proper was assigned to the broader category 'ideational
insanity', together with mania, general paralysis, dementia, and idiocy.[91]
In 1879, a third revised edition of the second half of *The Physiology
and Pathology of the Mind* was published as a separate volume entitled
The Pathology of Mind.[92] Like many of his peers, Maudsley noted the
difficulties arising when attempting to categorise mental disease correctly
and maintained that, for the time being, a system whereby illnesses were
divided according to symptoms rather than their 'real nature' was, while
provisional, necessary for practical reasons, in order to make the process
of diagnosing patients less complex and laborious.[93] When observing
patients in the asylum, Maudsley argued, the most striking contrast in
terms of symptoms was that between mania and melancholia, which

could be further divided into 'general' and 'partial', the latter suggesting that 'the intellectual disorder is limited to a few ideas'.[94] He suggested that this separation of insanity, with the third addition of general paralysis, corresponded to the traditional symptomatologic division that could be found in the work of Esquirol. These three types were, Maudsley remarked, discernible even to the untrained eye of a layman. However, upon closer examination of an asylum population the medical expert would soon discover a more complex and rich picture. Most importantly, one would not be able to escape the fact that in many lunatics the mental disease was one in which any intellectual derangement, even of the partial kind, was wholly absent. The skilled observer would find that such forms of madness where emotion was only or primarily affected were by far the most common; indeed, Maudsley went so far as to suggest that 'the affective disorder has been the fundamental trouble in almost all cases that have not been produced at once by direct physical injury'.[95] Thus, he reaffirmed his previous assertion from 1867, when he had cautioned his peers against the dangers of failing to recognise disorders of affect as proper forms of madness.[96]

Maudsley had made some changes to his nosology from previous editions, but maintained the separation between 'affective' and 'ideational' insanity, to which a third umbrella category, 'amentia', was added. Both melancholia and mania were placed in the second category of ideational insanity together with monomania and dementia, whereas affective insanity contained only two subclasses, 'instinctive' and 'moral'. Impulses to commit suicide were, Maudsley argued, particularly common in forms of madness where only the affective life was disordered, and was presented as closely related to homicidal and other destructive impulses.

The classification system presented in the 1879 edition of *The Pathology of Mind* had a strong air of a work in progress about it. Maudsley suggested as much himself, stating that 'I might abolish the division of affective insanity altogether, and place the varieties belonging to it under mania and melancholia, dividing these respectively into mania with delusion, and mania without delusion, and into melancholia with or without delusion'.[97] However, while he remained formally equivocal on whether or not melancholia should be classified as a single disease entity, he nevertheless proceeded to award an entire chapter to this form of insanity, a significant change from previous editions of the textbook. In a fourth edition of *The Pathology of Mind* published in 1895 Maudsley's nosology was revised in much the same way as anticipated, with the result that melancholia—particularly in its simple, non-delusional form—received more attention than any other form of madness.[98]

A comparatively strong focus on non-delusional melancholia was already apparent in the 1879 edition, where Maudsley suggested that it commonly appeared as the first stage of the disease, and sometimes persisted for the duration of illness. While the absence of delusion meant that the patient was able to conduct rational thought processes, their mental state would become 'profoundly changed notwithstanding: his feelings regarding persons and events are strangely perverted, so that impressions which would naturally be agreeable are painful'.[99] One of the most difficult aspects of melancholia for those who suffered from it, Maudsley argued, was the fact that the morbid feelings and ideas appeared so wholly unnatural and without reason, and often seemed to the patient's mind to have appeared quite suddenly, as if from out of thin air. For this reason, he argued, the melancholic patient would often draw the conclusion that the mental suffering had supernatural causes, as a form of divine retribution. However, the patient's belief that the emotional suffering was in response to having committed 'the unpardonable sin' had, Maudsley argued, a medical explanation. Morbid ideas and emotions might appear to arise 'spontaneously' as if they were conjured up by 'the suggestion of an evil spirit', but in actual fact they were the result of a traceable physiological process:

There is, first, a possible organic suggestion coming from a particular organ of the body in consequence of the special sympathies which the brain has with the different organs; secondly, there is that constant unconscious mental operation – more active perhaps when the brain is in an abnormal state – whereby the revival of latent ideas and feelings frequently takes place without our being able to give any account of it; thirdly, impressions from without, which seem so trivial as to be hardly noticed at the time, may still have their effects upon the mind, and, when the brain functions are disordered and overclouded by gloomy feeling, may be worked up into strange morbid ideas; and lastly, an idea may be excited sympathetically by another idea to which it has no apparent relation, particularly in a morbid brain, just as the muscles may notably be sympathetically excited sometimes by the contraction of certain other muscles with which they have no normal functional connection.[100]

Maudsley agreed with Clouston's remark that melancholic patients, while often able to think rationally, were not aware of the correct source of their altered mental state, and this was in itself one of the most difficult aspects of this disease, Maudsley suggested. Because melancholics were often able to think quite clearly and engage in rational conversation, their simultaneous inability to explicate their own apparently irrational suffering constituted a tremendous source of despair.[101] This was also one of the main reasons why they were often driven to suicide. The key to understanding suicide lay, Maudsley argued, in 'the instinctive love of life', which he held up as the 'real effective force against suicide'. This instinct was built into the constitution of each individual in the same way as the automated actions 'of the heart and of respiration'. Following from this, suicidal tendencies were evidence that 'the organic element' of the melancholic sufferer was 'so wanting in this fundamental quality that it could not assimilate and increase, but must be assimilated and decrease'.[102] In this way, the apparent contradiction of suicidality in melancholic patients suffering from religious delusions could be explained. It might seem 'curiously inconsistent', Maudsley remarked, that a person who perceives their mental suffering to be the result of having sinned against God and who fears 'eternal damnation' should be driven towards the very outcome they fear the most and which they believe is the cause of their suffering. This showed, he argued, that 'nature' was 'deeper and stronger than creed', driving the melancholic towards suicide 'by an impulse whose roots go far down below any conscious motive'.[103] This observation would later lead Maudsley to suggest that people suffering from simple or non-delusional melancholia were the most likely to commit suicide, and that such individuals were able to arrive at the decision through rational deliberation, as the only evident solution to intolerable mental pain and depression.

Towards a Standardised Diagnosis

In the last quarter of the century melancholia was solidified and homogenised chiefly in two ways. On the one hand, biomedical explanatory frameworks for mental disease were the norm for British physicians in the second half of the century, and in this context variations on physiological reconstitutions of melancholia as 'disordered emotion' were widely adopted. On the other hand, the range of symptoms listed was more focussed with less variation in the terminology used by different physicians. While earlier conceptions of melancholia were arguably more coherent and unified than descriptions of other forms of madness, the symptoms described by medical writers and the language used in such descriptions exhibited a far greater degree of idiosyncrasy than those of the late Victorian period. This shift was particularly pronounced in the nosological sections of textbooks on mental disease, and in published journal articles. But much is also revealed in the language used in patient journals and other asylum records, as well as in the case studies physicians liked to attach as illustrations to their nosological writings. However, as will be seen below and in the next chapter, the unifying symptom terms that were increasingly deployed in late nineteenth-century Victorian literature functioned in different ways. Mental pain and depression were both symptoms emphasised as defining features of melancholia in nosological writings, but the former rarely featured in case studies involving direct descriptions of individual patients' mental states. Its chief usefulness can be seen as streamlining diagnostic criteria for the purpose of textbook descriptions of melancholia; in other words, mental pain served as an umbrella term, a sort of professional shorthand, for a multitude of different expressions of distress and suffering.

In the last two decades of the century, case studies of melancholia made regular appearances in medical journals (particularly the *Journal of Mental Science*). Suicidal tendencies were frequently highlighted as a key symptom, such as in an article by one of Thomas Clouston's assistant physicians at Morningside in Edinburgh. Recounting a case of 'profound' and 'suicidal' melancholia, Carlyle Johnstone described the patient, a forty-year-old woman, who was admitted after a period of insanity lasting 'several weeks'. The patient's history, as derived from her medical certificate, suggested that she had been 'threatening to commit suicide' and 'had taken very little food'. Overall, '[h]er mental condition was one of profound depression', she was described as anxious and agitated and 'exclaiming that she was lost'. After several months in the asylum, she was still considered to exhibit suicidal tendencies, she reportedly stated on several occasions that 'she wants to be killed', and 'attempted to commit suicide' a number of times while on the ward.[104]

In a case of 'melancholia followed by monomania of exaltation', a twenty-nine-year-old woman was equally described as 'suicidal', with the propensity chiefly brought on by religious delusions: 'She felt that she was doomed to everlasting punishment'.[105] A forty-year-old woman was admitted to the pauper asylum in Worcester in a state of 'acute melancholia'. Several 'superficial scratches' to the skin were found on her body, believed to have been 'self-inflicted with suicidal intent'. She claimed to have inserted a needle into her stomach 'with the object of taking her life', but none was discovered upon examination. The author noted that she continued to be 'very suicidally inclined' until she eventually died, presumed to be suffering from phthisis. During the autopsy, a needle was discovered buried in her abdomen.[106] Twin sisters were admitted to the Warwick County Asylum in 1900, and were both diagnosed with melancholia upon admission. Arthur Wilcox, head physician at the hospital, described them both as having 'the same dominant delusion, viz., that she herself was the most wicked woman alive and was unfit to live, and both attempted suicide just before admission'.[107]

George Savage described a similar case of a young woman who was admitted to Bethlem after a brief melancholic episode reportedly triggered by the birth of her child. As her mental state deteriorated, 'she became suicidal and violent, refused food, said she was inhumanely wicked, that she has ruined her husband, and ought to be got rid of'.[108] Savage wrote extensively on melancholia in his major textbook, *Insanity and Allied Neuroses*, which was published in several editions from the mid-1880s onward, and paid particular attention to suicidal tendencies in melancholic patients. In addition to a handful of monographs, he was a regular contributor to the *Journal of Mental Science* (which he also co-edited with Daniel Hack Tuke between 1878 and 1892) as well as general medical journals.[109] In the first (1884) edition of his textbook, Savage regretfully noted that the physiological basis of mental disease was at present poorly understood. At the same time, he was optimistic that it was only a matter of time until the microscopic functions of the brain would be revealed to medical scientists.[110] Like Maudsley, he argued that at present the different forms of mental disease must be organised and described according to their external manifestations. He did, however, envisage a time when mental disorders could be classified 'according to the physiological changes which take place in the nerve centres'. While certain forms of insanity resulted in observable structural changes to brain tissue, other forms 'depend for their origin on the existence of some bodily defect or degeneration, which, causing irritation at the periphery, in the end sets up brain disease by a continuity of the nervous tissues, or by some other reflective process'.[111]

Thus, while Savage expressed greater reservations about what physiological research could presently reveal about the internal nervous operations of people believed to suffer from mental disease, he nevertheless recognised the prevailing model for explicating disordered mental functions. While advising his readers that 'the pathological basis of melancholia' remained, as yet, uncertain, it appeared that the disease could be attributed to 'impaired nutrition of the nervous centres and the conducting system'.[112] Savage offered the following descriptive summary of melancholia:

> Melancholia is a state of mental depression, in which the misery is unreasonable either in relation to its apparent cause, or in the peculiar form it assumes, the mental pain depending on physical and bodily changes, and not directly on the environment.[113]

On the pathology and aetiology of the disease, Savage explained that the 'mental pain' in melancholia could be the result of 'change in the nutrition of the brain depending on some general or local disease', but equally this 'disordered process' could occur through the 'nervous system' becoming exhausted.[114] In addition to these possible origins, Savage warned that 'any cause, bodily or mental, which worries the body or mind, any cause which by its constancy, or by its frequent repetition, gives no chance of repair, may also cause melancholia'.[115] Thus, Savage equally allowed for the idea, put forward by Griesinger, Laycock, and others, that morbid cerebral action could be triggered by negative thoughts alone.

As the works discussed above illustrate, towards the end of the century the melancholia diagnosis was increasingly coherent and standardised, coalescing around four key symptoms: depression, suicidal tendencies, mental pain, and religious delusions. The focus on suicidality also facilitated another development that would have profound and lasting consequences for the ways in which psychiatric knowledge is brought to bear upon emotional states. The suicidal impulse was often seen as strongest in people suffering from simple, or non-delusional, melancholia, as they were able to reason about their suffering. This meant that physicians were increasingly concerned with this milder form of the disorder, which sat uneasily on the border between sanity and insanity. In this way, a final key development in the reconceptualisation of melancholia as a modern biomedical disorder, and a precursor to twentieth-century depression, occurred: the expansion of the realm of psychiatric knowledge to include emotional states not considered strictly pathological.

OBSCURING THE BOUNDARY BETWEEN NORMAL
AND PATHOLOGICAL EMOTIONS

As noted in Chapter 4, Griesinger had argued for early intervention to prevent melancholics from deteriorating into more severe forms of insanity. This argument was echoed by British physicians in the last quarter of the century. George Savage emphasised that early diagnosis and treatment of melancholia was imperative. In its simple form, which often constituted the early stages of illness, melancholia might not manifest as a full-blown mental disorder; in some cases it was only distinguishable by 'slight perversions of feeling and intellect of a gloomy nature'. However, echoing Griesinger, Savage argued that it was of 'the utmost importance' that even this mild form or stage of the disease was recognised as pathological and that patients gain access to diagnostics and treatment. If simple melancholia was not properly acknowledged, the disorder 'may become chronic and incurable'.[116] Treatment and confinement was also important for another reason—to prevent melancholics from committing suicide. Despite his sceptical stance towards statistics on suicidal patients noted above, Savage held that one of the most significant features of melancholia was the frequency with which its sufferers exhibited suicidal tendencies. He suggested that the suicidal propensity could arise from a number of causes, some of which were associated with delusions, particularly of a religious kind. However, while patients suffering from other forms of insanity were sometimes known to attempt or commit suicide, such instances were often accidental, whereas 'suicide must ever be looked upon as one of the dangerous symptoms connected chiefly with melancholia'.[117]

William Bevan Lewis also noted the problem of suicidal intent in non-delusional melancholics, who were able to reason about their suffering and search in vain for a rational cause. As medical director at the Wakefield Asylum in West Riding, Yorkshire, and successor to the famous neurologist James Crichton-Browne, Lewis readily embraced a biomedical model for melancholia. This can at least in part be attributed to the context in which he worked; at West Riding there was a significant focus on cerebral post-mortem examinations and diagnostics were constituted within a solid biological framework.[118] His commitment to neurology and neurophysiology was in strong evidence in his textbook, which commenced with a substantial section on anatomy and histology, made up of several detailed chapters on the various parts of the brain and spinal cord. He went on to describe simple melancholia as 'forms of a purely emotional or affec-tive insanity, where there is mental pain or emotional distress apart from obvious intellectual disturbance'.[119] It was not, however, the intensity of the mental pain that set it apart from similar feelings in healthy individ-uals, but rather its cause. If 'the mental pain is the result of trivial exciting agencies, if moral or physical agencies arouse emotional states out of all proportion to what would occur in a healthy mind, then we infer that the grey cortex of the brain is so far disordered as to functionate abnormally, and we speak of the result as pathological depression'.[120]

Lewis quoted Griesinger on the topic of mental pain as a '"dispropor-tionately excessive" reaction' in melancholia, suggesting that '[e]motional disturbances as the result of disease differ from the normal reactions of health, not only in volume, but also in nature'. Drawing upon Herbert Spencer's psychology, Lewis went on to suggest that part of the problem lay in 'pain' being a 'non-relational' emotion. This meant that it could not easily coexist with other emotional states, making it difficult to esti-mate 'the degree of mental alienation in melancholia'.[121] This perceived inability to deduce the extent of the melancholic patient's psychological pain and deterioration made the threat of suicide all the more insid-ious. He suggested, however, that because patients were often capable of rational thought, they struggled to resist their suicidal propensities.[122]

This tension between rational thought and emotional pain in suicidal melancholics was discussed in detail by Charles Mercier in his *Sanity and Insanity* (1890). A consulting physician on mental disease at Charing Cross Hospital in London, Mercier encountered melancholic patients outside the asylum walls, and paid particular attention to suicidality in melancholic sufferers in the earlier, non-delusional stages of the disease. He alerted his readers to the 'tendency to suicide' that was a common feature of melancholia, and went on to emphasise the unnaturalness of self-inflicted death. 'Suicide', he argued, 'is so complete and violent a reversal of the strongest and most fundamental of instincts – the instinct of self-preservation – that its origin, and the frequency of its occurrence, are extremely puzzling'.[123] However, when describing this phenomenon in melancholic patients, Mercier offered an explanation for the apparent enigma of suicide. With a nod to the growing body of non-medical research on the causes and prevalence of suicide in Europe, he observed that suicides were clearly committed by sane individuals in many cases, and could result from of a host of factors, such as financial troubles or unrequited love. In light of this knowledge, Mercier suggested that the way out of a misery which is autogenetic, and does not correspond with or depend on adversity of circumstances, may be the same as that out of a misery, the same degree, which is justified by the circumstances in which the organism is placed. There may be no justification in his circumstances for the misery which the melancholy man experiences, but his misery is as acute, as real, as profound as that of the man whose circumstances are extremely adverse; nay, there is no such misery as that of melancholia; and under the pressure of this feeling suicide may be the natural and quasi-normal course to take. Here, then, a large class of suicidal cases receives an explanation on grounds which import no new principle of action into human motives, and which harmonize with the general course of human nature.[124]

While suicidal intent may in a healthy individual arise from organism–environment interaction where an adverse event might trigger a desire to commit suicide, in melancholic patients a similar kind of event would occur internally, with the diseased mental state itself, rather than some external cause, producing the adverse reaction. In this way, from the argument that suicide was the antithesis of the fundamental evolutionary principle—the organism's struggle for self-preservation—Mercier arrived at the conclusion that when held against the pain and misery of melancholia, suicide would in fact appear as a natural act and a reasonable solution to intolerable suffering.

Maudsley arrived at much the same view a couple of years later. In an article entitled 'Suicide in Simple Melancholy', which appeared in the *Medical Magazine* in 1892, he presented a narrative of melancholic suffering that was much revised from his earlier published work on the disease. Maudsley's choice of word is important to note—the use of 'melancholy' rather than the medical 'melancholia' speaks to an emphasis on the very early stages of the disease, when the sufferer's state of mind was not yet disordered to such an extent that one might speak of insanity proper. Yet, like Savage, Maudsley firmly maintained that this condition warranted medical attention, primarily due to the often overwhelming desire to commit suicide in such individuals. Indeed, he suggested that the suicidal propensity was as a rule much more intense, persistent, and ultimately more dangerous than in people suffering from melancholia proper. In the latter, suicidal thoughts might plague the patient for years before any action would be taken, whereas the simple melancholic was far more likely to end their life swiftly.[125]

Why was this so? It was not the case, Maudsley argued, that the pain was more intense in simple melancholy than in melancholia proper. Rather, the problem lay in the fact that, in the absence of any intellectual derangement, the individual was able to reason about their condition and thus fully appreciate the absurdity and hopelessness of such misery without apparent cause. It was this absence of any traceable external circumstances to explain the mental pain that marked this state of mind as disordered, despite the patient being otherwise 'sane'. If such misery was caused by 'misfortune, bereavement, soured hope, disdained love, crosses or losses in business, or other sufficient blow to self-love or self-interest', then the reaction was to be considered normal, and the individual would soon recover. However, if the suffering arose 'due to internal failure of the springs of re-action, without external cause or in measure and duration out of all proportion to such cause as there may have been, then it is morbid'.[126]

The mental pain of simple melancholics was consequently of a particularly excruciating kind. They would find themselves able to take in their surroundings and engage with the world, yet feeling utterly trapped in a permanent state of emotional suffering:

> Sane enough to feel keenly what they suffer and to contrast their woeful deadness with the joyous energy around them, crushed to despair by the serene continuity of things in contrast with the discontinuity of their interest in them, in the world but not of it, sufferers not doers – they cannot bear the burden of a wretched existence.[127]

For such persons, then, '[o]ne way of escape alone suggests itself, dim and undefined in his mind and shrunk from with horror at first, but viewed more nearly and clearly when he feels his anguish too great to be borne longer: it is suicide'.[128] Thus, in simple melancholy the unnatural act of suicide appeared as the only natural solution to intolerable suffering. Following from this, Maudsley argued that upon examination every suicide could be found to have an 'explanatory' cause. In cases of non-delusional melancholy, the expounding factor was unequivocally clear:

> Suicide of this sort, springing from suffering that is intolerable, is natural in motive and logical in fact, whatever may be thought of it from a moral standpoint: the outcome in consciousness of the sum of the despair of

the life-lacking organic elements, it is a supreme, final and (if we may use the word in this connection) fit act of adjustment to the outer world with which the individual can no longer contend. It is the remedy for the malady of life which has become insupportable.[129]

Such an unambiguous rationalisation of suicide is noteworthy even for a medical scientist of Maudsley's convictions.[130] Within a philosophy of mind firmly rooted in an evolutionary paradigm, suicide resulting from the internal conflict of melancholic suffering could nevertheless be construed as natural and logical. Indeed, it was precisely the conflict between each organism's desire for self-preservation and the profound mental pain of simple melancholy that allowed the suicidal propensity to arise with such force and intensity. '[W]here the love of life is struggling against its ebb', Maudsley warned, 'the misery is the greatest and the danger most urgent'.[131]

While the *Medical Magazine* article referred to the condition as 'simple melancholy' and emphasised its ambiguous status in relation to insanity proper, a few years later Maudsley reworked the article to fit into a chapter on melancholia in the final, much revised, edition of *The Pathology of Mind* (1895). This version of the textbook contained two, significantly expanded, chapters devoted to melancholia, including a comprehensive section on 'simple melancholia'. This largely mirrored the article on 'Suicide in Simple Melancholy', with a notable modification being the use of 'melancholia' in place of 'melancholy'. Maudsley described this milder form of melancholia proper as 'a class of cases of mental depression' where 'there is neither delusion nor actual disorder of thought'. He maintained that such conditions were not melancholia 'in strict sense, since there is no real derangement of mind', rather in these states there was 'only a profound pain of mind paralysing its functions – an essential *psychalgia*'.[132]

While in the 1860s Maudsley had issued a sharp caution against the failure to properly recognise non-delusional, affective disorders of mind as forms of true madness, three decades later he arrived at a conclusion that appears, at first glance, to contradict his former argument. However, what we are witnessing here is the infancy of a process whereby medico-psychological (and later psychiatric) attention was increasingly brought to bear upon aspects of the human emotional and cognitive life that were *not* considered to be states of insanity in the proper sense.[133] It is not possible within the scope of this book to address this important shift in how post-nineteenth-century medical psychologists and psychiatrists would constitute the relationship between human emotion, behaviour, and pathology. However, the implications of Maudsley's revision of his earlier argument must not be overlooked. The decision to award significant attention in a textbook on mental pathology to the description and analysis of an emotional state which by his own account was not a form of disease, was, while perhaps more subtly done, nonetheless at least as critical a revolution in medical thinking as the early nineteenth-century argument that some forms of madness were chiefly of the affective kind.

CONCLUSION

This chapter has mapped the key ways in which melancholia as was modernised and standardised in the final decades of the nineteenth century. Through this process, the diagnosis came to centre upon four key symptoms: depression, suicidal tendencies, mental pain, and religious delusions. It is important to note, however, that the developments described here were neither universal nor did they occur in a simple, linear fashion. Biomedical ways of explaining the mind continued to rely in some instances on terminology and concepts that pre-dated nineteenth-century experimental physiology. Much like psychiatry today, Victorian medical psychologists struggled to make sense of the mind in strictly scientific terms, and despite their strong epistemological commitment to biomedicine, they were forced to make use of other tools in order to carry out many of the practical aspects of their work. In particular, physiological explanations of mental operations were of little use when it came to diagnosing patients arriving at the asylum or hospital. Here, observable and communicated 'symptoms' provided the major source of information about which type of disease physicians were faced with. However, the symptoms described in this chapter were not, as a rule, communicated as such by the patients. The intellectual work required to turn the chaos of human emotions that met physicians on the asylum wards into recordable, classifiable symptoms was thus considerable. The uneasy relationship between what was observed, communicated, recorded, and published is the focus of the next chapter, which traces melancholia as a diagnosis on its journey between the casebook and the textbook.

NOTES

1. John Charles Bucknill, "The Diagnosis of Insanity," *Journal of Mental Science* 2 (1856): 229.

2. Roger Smith, *Being Human: Historical Knowledge and the Creation of Human Nature* (Manchester: Manchester University Press, 2007), 122.

3. George H. Savage, *Insanity and Allied Neuroses: Practical and Clinical* (London: Cassell, 1884), 12.

4. Savage, *Insanity*, 12. Such concerns have persisted in psychiatry, most recently voiced in response to the fifth edition of the *DSM*. See the Conclusion of this book.

5. Thomas S. Clouston, *Clinical Lectures on Mental Diseases* (London: J. & A. Churchill, 1883), 112.

6. *An Act (8 & 9 Vict. c. 100) for the Regulation of the Care and Treatment of Lunatics*, 1845, Schedule D, Section 46: "Order for the Reception of a Pauper Patient".

7. Thomas N. Brushfield, "On Medical Certificates of Insanity," *The Lancet* 115 (1880): 712.

8. Edwin S. Schneidman, *Suicide as Psychache: A Clinical Approach to Self-Destructive Behavior* (Plymouth: Rowman and Littlefield, 1993), 51.

9. E.g. Clouston, *Clinical Lectures*; Richard von Krafft-Ebing, *Die Melancholie: Eine klinische Studie* (Erlangen: Ferdinand Enke, 1874); Henry Maudsley, *The Pathology of Mind: A Study of Its Distempers, Deformities, and Disorders*, 4th ed. (London: Macmillan, 1895).

10. See e.g. Steven Mee, et al., "Psychological Pain: A Review of Evidence," *Journal of Psychiatric Research* 40, No. 8 (2006): 680–690; Israel Orbach, et al., "Mental Pain and Its Relationship to Suicidality and Life Meaning," *Suicide and Life-Threatening Behaviour* 30, No. 3 (2003): 231–241.

11. See the Introduction and Chapter 3 for discussions on differing meanings of this term in the Victorian period and the present.

12. *Diagnostic and Statistical Manual for Mental Disorders, Fifth Edition (DSM-5)* (Washington, DC: The American Psychiatric Association, 2013), 161; *International Statistical Classification of Diseases and Related Health Problems, 10th Revision (ICD-10)*, World Health Organisation, 2010, section F32 ("Depressive Episode"), http://apps.who.int/classifications/icd10/browse/2010/en#/F32 (last accessed 08/05/2013).

13. See e.g. Savage, *Insanity*, 151; Griesinger, *Die Pathologie und Therapie*, 213; Clouston, *Clinical Lectures*, 32; William Bevan Lewis, *A Text-Book of Mental Diseases*, 2nd ed. (London: Charles Griffin, 1899), 115.

14. See e.g. Samuel Smiles' Victorian bestseller: Samuel Smiles, *Self-Help, with Illustrations of Character and Conduct* (John Murray: London, 1859).

15. Maudsley, *Physiology and Pathology of the Mind*, 322.
16. Henry Monro, *Remarks on Insanity: Its Nature and Treatment* (London: John Churchill, 1851), 1.
17. *A Bill to Regulate the Care and Treatment of Insane Persons*, House of Commons, Session 1828 (78), Vol. I.323.
18. As decreed by a parliamentary Act of that year: *Licensed Lunatic Asylums: A bill for amending the Laws Relating to Houses Licensed by the Metropolitan Commissioners and Justices of the Peace for the Reception of Insane Persons*, House of Commons, Session 1842, Vol. III.113.
19. *Report of the Metropolitan Commissioners in Lunacy to the Lord Chancellor, Presented to Both Houses of Parliament by Command of Her Majesty* (London: Bradbury & Evans, 1844), 178–179.
20. The Victorian fascination with numbers (mirrored in much of nineteenth-century Europe) was the focus of a conference organised by the British Association for Victorian Studies, held at Royal Holloway in London. A full list of speakers and papers can be found here: http://bavs2013.wordpress.com/programme/ (last accessed 03/08/2013).
21. Elis Malmeström, *Carl von Linné: Geniets kamp för klarhet* (Stockholm: Bonniers, 1964), 66.
22. Michel Foucault, *The Order of Things: An Archaeology of the Human Sciences* (London: Routledge, 2002 [1966]), 144.
23. Geoffrey C. Bowker and Susan Leigh Star, *Sorting Things Out: Classification and Its Consequences* (London: The MIT Press, 1999), 17.
24. On the emergence of medical statistics, see Eileen Magnello and Ann Hardy, eds., *The Road to Medical Statistics* (Amsterdam and New York: Rodopi, 2002).
25. Terrence D. Murphy, "Medical Knowledge and Statistical Methods in Early Nineteenth-Century France," *Medical History* 25 (1981): 303–304.
26. Murphy, Statistical Methods, 305.
27. Murphy, Statistical Methods, 307–308.
28. Elaine Murphy, "The Administration of Insanity in England 1800 to 1870," in *The Confinement of the Insane: International Perspectives, 1800–1965*, eds. Roy Porter and David Wright (Cambridge: Cambridge University Press, 2003), 337.
29. David Wright, "The Certification of Insanity in Nineteenth-Century England and Wales," *History of Psychiatry* 9 (1998): 272–274.
30. *An Act (8 & 9 Vict. c. 100) for the Regulation of the Care and Treatment of Lunatics*, House of Commons, No. 373, Vol. IV.181, 1845; *Lunacy Asylums and Pauper Lunatics. A Bill to Amend the Law Concerning Lunatic Asylums, and the Care of Pauper Lunatics in England*, House of Commons, No. 358, Vol. IV.7, 1845.
31. Wright, "The Certification of Insanity," 274.

32. A similar body, the 'Board of Commissioners,' was set up for Scotland the following decade. *An Act (20 & 21 Victoria c. 71) for the Regulation of the Care and Treatment of Lunatics, and for the Provision, Maintenance, and Regulation of Lunatic Asylums in Scotland*, 25 August, 1857.
33. Lunacy Commission, Circular Letters, Letter no. 69, May 7, 1857, The National Archives, Kew, Ref: MH51/236.
34. Lunacy Commission, Circular Letters, Letter no. 127, February 5, 1870, The National Archives, Kew, Ref: MH51/237.
35. *Care and Treatment of Lunatics Act*, Schedule (D.), Section 48.
36. Under Scottish law, two certificates were required for both private and pauper patients.
37. These templates underwent minor modifications with subsequent amendments of the Lunacy Act in 1853 and 1862.
38. *Care and Treatment of Lunatics Act*, Section 51.
39. While Scottish asylum physicians operated under a separate lunacy law and reported to their own Board of Commissioners, the result was largely the same in terms of the kind of statistics produced.
40. Another body created by the 1845 Acts; a group of appointed judges and physicians whose task it was to carry out regular 'visitations' of the asylums in their jurisdiction. Their findings and recommendations were included in the annual report of each asylum.
41. *Care and Treatment of Lunatics Act*, Section 60. Italics removed.
42. Lunacy Commission, *Circular Letters*, Letter no. 7, 19 January 1846, The National Archives, Kew, Ref: MH51/236.
43. Eric J. Engstrom, *Clinical Psychiatry in Imperial Germany: A History of Psychiatric Practice* (Ithaca, NY: Cornell University Press, 2004), 35–44.
44. "Proceedings at the Annual Meeting of the Medico-Psychological Association, held at the Royal College of Physicians, on Thursday, July 13th, 1865," *Journal of Mental Science* 11 (1865): 402–407.
45. "Proceedings at the Annual Meeting of the Medico-Psychological Association, held at the Royal College of Physicians, on Wednesday, July 31st, 1867," *Journal of Mental Science* 13 (1867): 402–403.
46. The Commission moreover took measures to ensure that the new tables were implemented by sending out a reminder to all asylum superintendents in 1870. See Lunacy Commission, *Circular Letters*, Letter no. 126, 3 February 1870, The National Archives, Kew, Ref: MH 51/237.
47. *Twentieth Annual Report of the Commissioners in Lunacy to the Lord Chancellor*, House of Commons, June 4, 1866, 44–46.
48. "Proceedings" (1867), 410.
49. Henry Maudsley, *The Pathology of Mind*, 3rd ed. (London: Macmillan, 1879), 296.
50. Maudsley, *The Pathology of Mind*, 3rd ed., 327.

51. Savage, *Insanity*, 12.
52. Lunacy Commission, *Circular Letters*, Letter no. 156, 20 February 1876, The National Archives, Kew, Ref: MH51/237.
53. This is based on a survey of statistics and casebooks from the following asylums: Parkside (Cheshire), Brookwood (Surrey), Hanwell (Sussex), Bethlem (London), Morningside (Edinburgh), and Ticehurst (Sussex).
54. For a more in-depth discussion of this process, see Åsa Jansson, "From Statistics' to Diagnostics: Medical Certificates, Melancholia, and 'Suicidal Propensities' in Victorian Psychiatry," *Journal of Social History* 46, No. 3 (2013): 716–731.
55. See also e.g. W.F. Farquharson, "On Melancholia: An Analysis of 730 Consecutive Cases," *Journal of Mental Science* 40, No. 169 (1894): 196–206.
56. Thomas N. Brushfield, "Report of the Medical Superintendent for the Year 1854," in *Annual Report of the Committee of Visitors to the Cheshire County Lunatic Asylum* (Chester: Evans and Gresty, 1855).
57. Olive Anderson's study sheds light on the vexing questions facing physicians who were expected to care for 'suicidal' lunatics. See Olive Anderson, *Suicide in Victorian and Edwardian England* (Oxford: Clarendon Press, 1987), 402–405.
58. Lunacy Commission, *Circular Letters*, Letter dated 21 March 1877, The National Archives, Kew, Ref: MH51/237.
59. George Savage, "Constant Watching of Suicidal Cases," *Journal of Mental Science* 30 (1884): 17–19.
60. Savage, 'Constant Watching', 17.
61. 'Proceedings' (1865), 415.
62. 'Proceedings' (1865), 417.
63. Bucknill had also voiced concerns about the format of medical certificates a few years earlier. John Charles Bucknill, "On Medical Certificates of Insanity," *Journal of Mental Science* 7 (1860): 79–88.
64. Thomas N. Brushfield, "Report of the Medical Superintendent for the Year 1870," in *Annual Report of the Committee of Visitors to the Surrey County Lunatic Asylum at Brookwood* (London: Batten & Davies, 1871), 21–22.
65. Brushfield, 'On Medical Certificates', 712.
66. Brushfield, 'On Medical Certificates', 712.
67. Brushfield, 'On Medical Certificates', 712.
68. Bowker and Star, *Sorting Things Out*, 24.
69. This tension has been the focus of much scholarly attention. See for instance Frank Turner, "The Victorian Conflict between Science and Religion," *Isis* 69 (1978): 356–376; Geoffrey Cantor, Thomas Dixon, and Stephen Pumfrey, eds., *Science and Religion: New Historical Perspectives* (Cambridge: Cambridge University Press, 2010).

70. See for instance: Esther Cohen, *The Modulated Scream: Pain in Medieval Culture* (Chicago: Chicago University Press, 2009); John R. Yamamoto-Wilson, *Pain, Pleasure, and Perversity: Discourses of Suffering in Seventeenth Century England* (Farnham: Ashgate, 2013); Jan Frans van Dijkhuizen and Karl A.E. Enenkel, eds., *The Sense of Suffering: Constructions of Physical Pain in Early Modern Culture* (Leiden: Brill, 2009).

71. See for instance the special issue of *Interdisciplinary Studies in the Long Nineteenth Century* on 'Perspectives on Pain' (No. 15, 2012). See also Andrew Hodgkiss, *From Lesion to Metaphor: Chronic Pain in British, French and German Medical Writings, 1800–1914* (Amsterdam: Rodopi, 2000); Joanna Bourke, "Pain, Sympathy, and the Medical Encounter between the Mid Eighteenth and the Mid Twentieth Centuries," *Historical Research* 85, No. 229 (2012): 430–452.

72. Javier Moscoso, *Pain: A Cultural History* (Basingstoke: Palgrave Macmillan, 2012), 106.

73. Astell is primarily known as an early advocate of women's education. See Joan Kinnaird, "Mary Astell and the Conservative Contribution to English Feminism," *Journal of British Studies* 19, No. 1 (1979–80): 53–75.

74. Mary Astell, "Letter V: To Mr. Norris," in *Letters Concerning the Love of God, between the Author of the Proposal to the Ladies, and Mr. John Norris*, eds. John Norris (London: Manship and Wilkin, 1705), 53.

75. Richard Fiddes, *Fifty Two Practical Discourses on Several Subjects, Six of Which Were Never Before Published* (London: Wyat, Took, Barber, and Clements, 1720), 639.

76. Cf. Emma Sutton on William James' perception of evil: "When Misery and Physics Collide: William James on 'the Problem of Evil'," *Medical History* 55, No. 3 (2011): 389–392.

77. Eighteenth-century medical works played an important part in fusing spiritual and scientific language. See e.g. David Hartley on mental pain in *Observations on Man, His Frame, His Duty, and His Expectations*, 4th ed. (Warrington, Johnson and Eyres, 1810 [1751]), 263.

78. This is discussed in Chapter 2. See also Hodgkiss, *From Lesion to Metaphor*.

79. Griesinger, *Die Pathologie und Therapie*. Griesinger used the more literal term 'psychischen Schmerz' rather than 'Psychalgie'.

80. J.M. Schiff, *Lehrbuch des Physiologie des Menschen: I. Muskel- und Nervenphysiologie* (Lahr: Verlag von M. Schauenburg & Co, 1858–59).

81. Griesinger, *Die Pathologie und Therapie*, 34.

82. Griesinger, *Die Pathologie und Therapie*, 38. See also Maudsley, *Pathology of Mind*, 3rd ed., 360–361.

83. Maudsley, *The Pathology of Mind*, 3rd ed., 362.

84. See e.g. D. Denham, "The Forgiveness of All Sin, Except the Sin Against the Holy Ghost," *The Gospel Magazine* 1, No. 2 (1841): 50–53; H.O. "On The Unpardonable Sin," *The Christian Guardian and Church of England Magazine* (1833): 257–259; Ichabod Smith Spencer, *A Pastor's Sketches, or, Conversations with Curious Inquirers Respecting the Way of Salvation* (New York: M.W. Dodd, 1868), 323–329.

85. Henry Ward Beecher, *Sermons: No 1: Strength According to the Days* (London: J. Heaton & Son, 1864), 89–90.

86. Beecher, *Sermons*, 160.

87. Beecher, *Sermons*, 194.

88. Maudsley, *The Pathology of Mind*, 3rd ed., 360.

89. George Fielding Blandford, *Insanity and Its Treatment: Lectures on the Treatment, Medical and Legal, of Insane Patients*, 3rd ed. (New York: William Wood, 1886), 112.

90. Blandford, *Insanity and Its Treatment*, 142–143.

91. Henry Maudsley, *The Physiology and Pathology of the Mind* (London: Macmillan, 1867), 323. See Chapter 4 for details of Maudsley's earlier nosology.

92. Maudsley, *The Pathology of Mind*, 3rd ed. An independent third edition of *The Physiology of Mind* had been published three years previously: *The Physiology of Mind* (London: Macmillan, 1876).

93. Maudsley, *The Pathology of Mind*, 3rd ed., 297.

94. Maudsley, *The Pathology of Mind*, 3rd ed., 326.

95. Maudsley, *The Pathology of Mind*, 3rd ed., 328.

96. See Chapter 4.

97. Maudsley, *The Pathology of Mind*, 3rd ed., 329. Savage made a similar remark about his system, Savage, *Insanity*, 15.

98. See below.

99. Maudsley, *The Pathology of Mind*, 3rd ed., 358.

100. Maudsley, *The Pathology of Mind*, 3rd ed., 359–360.

101. Maudsley, *The Pathology of Mind*, 3rd ed., 358–359.

102. Maudsley, *The Pathology of Mind*, 3rd ed., 388.

103. Maudsley, *The Pathology of Mind*, 3rd ed., 385.

104. Carlyle Johnstone, "Case of Profound and Somewhat Prolonged Suicidal Melancholia; Diarrhaea with Fever; Recovery," *Journal of Mental Science* 31, No. 134 (1885): 203.

105. (author unknown), "Melancholia followed by Monomania of Exaltation," *Journal of Mental Science* 26, No. 116 (1881): 564.

106. G.M.P. Braine-Hartnell, "Acute Melancholia: Attempted Suicide by Inserting a Needle into the Abdomen. Death Nearly Thirteen Months After," *Journal of Mental Science* 39 (1893): 397–399.

107. Arthur W. Wilcox, "Insanity of Twins; Twins Suffering from Acute Melancholia," *Journal of Mental Science* 47, No. 197 (1901): 349. Of interest is also e.g. F.A. Elkins, "A Case of Melancholia: Sudden Illness and Death," *The Lancet* 141, No. 3633 (1893): 858; A.F. Mickle, "Insanity of Twins: Twins Suffering from Melancholia," *Journal of Mental Science* 30, No. 129 (1884): 67–74; J. Neil, "Three Cases of Recovery from Melancholia After Unusually Long Periods," *Journal of Mental Science* 41, No. 172 (1895): 86–89; A. Patton, "Two Cases of Melancholia," *Journal of Mental Science* 31, No. 136 (1886): 499–501.
108. Savage, *Insanity*, 1884.
109. Savage's status as something of a Victorian medical celebrity was epitomised by his inclusion in *Vanity Fair*'s 'Men of the Day' series in 1912. 'Men of the Day', *Vanity Fair* 1317 (1912).
110. Savage, *Insanity*, 9–10.
111. Savage, *Insanity*, 12–13.
112. Savage, *Insanity*, 130.
113. Savage, *Insanity*, 151.
114. On this aetiological point—the exhaustion of the nervous system—descriptions of melancholia did at times intersect with those of neurasthenia. See Chapter 4.
115. Savage, *Insanity*, 162–163.
116. Savage, *Insanity*, 167.
117. Savage, *Insanity*, 193–194.
118. Jennifer Wallis, "The Bones of the Insane," *History of Psychiatry* 24, No. 2 (2013): 196–211 and *Investigating the Body in the Victorian Asylum: Doctors, Patients, and Practices* (London: Palgrave Macmillan, 2017).
119. Lewis, *Mental Diseases*, 138.
120. Lewis, *Mental Diseases*, 115.
121. Lewis, *Mental Diseases*, 116.
122. Lewis, *Mental Diseases*, 140.
123. Charles A. Mercier, *Sanity and Insanity* (London: Walter Scott, 1890), 349.
124. Mercier, *Sanity and Insanity*, 350.
125. Henry Maudsley, "Suicide in Simple Melancholy," *Medical Magazine* 1 (1892): 48–57.
126. Maudsley, "Suicide in Simple Melancholy," 46.
127. Maudsley, "Suicide in Simple Melancholy," 48.
128. Maudsley, "Suicide in Simple Melancholy," 48.
129. Maudsley, "Suicide in Simple Melancholy," 49.
130. Cf. contemporaneous sociological views, esp. Durkheim's 'anomie' as a cause of suicide. Émile Durkheim, *Suicide: A Study in Sociology* (London: Routledge and Kegan Paul, 1952 [1897]).
131. Maudsley, "Suicide in Simple Melancholy," 51.

132. Maudsley, *The Pathology of Mind*, 4th ed., 167–168.
133. Another example of this was the increasing medical attention brought to bear upon 'minor' acts of 'self-mutilation' such as 'hair-plucking and face-picking' in this period, behaviours that were seen to occur in people suffering from mental disease, but which 'were also seen to blend seamlessly with the "nervous, fidgety, restless habits"' that were equally considered '"common among people who are not insane"'. Sarah Chaney, "Self-Control, Selfishness, and Mutilation: How Medical Is Self-Injury Anyway?" *Medical History* 55, No. 3 (2011): 380.

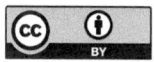

CHAPTER 6

Diagnosing Melancholia in the Victorian Asylum

A typical case of melancholia, as we shall see, runs a somewhat definite course, like a fever, and has often all the characters of an acute disease, in this being to the physician unlike a mere feeling of melancholy.[1]

Thomas S. Clouston (1883)

On 15 August 1874, a young doctor was admitted as a private patient into the Royal Edinburgh Asylum at Morningside. On the medical certificate and reception order that accompanied his arrival it was stated that the patient, Moses B., was 'suicidal'. The two certifying physicians testified that the patient had communicated to them a belief that his soul was lost. He was reported as having taken 'a poisonous dose of Belladonna', and his father and brother had seen it necessary to have him sent to the asylum since they felt that he could not 'be left alone' for the fear 'that he would seek to destroy himself'. Upon admission, the attending physician determined that his 'depression' was 'considerable', and made a note of his 'suicidal tendencies', which consisted in 'taking belladonna, refusing food, &c'. The patient's recent mental symptoms were listed as 'delusions such as that his soul is lost, that he ought to die, and thinks he is committing great sins'. He was given the diagnosis melancholia, with a special reference made to his persistent suicidal tendencies.[2]

© The Author(s) 2021
Å Jansson, *From Melancholia to Depression*,
Mental Health in Historical Perspective,
https://doi.org/10.1007/978-3-030-54802-5_6

Moses was what today might be referred to as a 'textbook case' of melancholia in the late-Victorian period: profound depression of mind, delusions of a religious nature, and persistent suicidal tendencies. Once inside the walls of Morningside, his case notes tell of repeated attempts by the patient to take his own life. Moses was considered such an exemplary case of melancholia that Joseph Brown, assisting physician at the asylum, proceeded to write up the case as an article for the *Edinburgh Medical Journal* later that year, presented as a typical case of 'suicidal melancholia' that served as a 'striking illustration of the great difficulty there exists in preventing a determined suicidal patient from accomplishing his object'.[3] According to Morningside's superintendent, Thomas Clouston, such cases were becoming increasingly common. In his annual report submitted that same year to the Board of Commissioners, the body overseeing the management of Scottish asylums, Clouston remarked that in 1874,

> [t]he number whose malady was characterised by depression of mind was most unusually large. I find no fewer than 88 under the head of Melancholia, a number greater by 70 per cent than the average number classified under that heading during the previous ten years, though, as we have seen, the excess of admissions this year was only 14 per cent. Many of the worst of these cases were more desperately intent on taking away their own lives than any patients I have ever had. The ingenuity, determination, and persistence of this suicidal propensity in some of them would scarcely be believed by any one who had not experienced it.[4]

The statistical tables accompanying the report confirmed Clouston's assessment: of the 88 melancholic patients admitted, 67 were listed as exhibiting 'suicidal tendencies'. It certainly appeared that an unusually large number of people suffered from melancholia in 1874, and that a significant majority were intent on taking their own lives. However, like many of his peers Clouston suggested that statistical tables did not necessarily represent a simple, discoverable truth. The Union of Chargeability Act[5] passed in the previous decade had made pauper lunatics in England and Wales chargeable to unions instead of single parishes, resulting in a rise in admissions of pauper patients in English asylums. This, Clouston argued, had been held up by a number of people 'as proof that lunacy was rapidly on the increase' across the border in the south, but in fact it 'merely shewed how the numbers of the registered insane were increased by an Act of Parliament'.[6]

When deploying Clouston's own reasoning to the statistics on melancholia, a similar picture could be seen to emerge. The increase in melancholic patients coincided with Clouston's appointment as superintendent of Morningside the previous year following the death of his predecessor, David Skae. This event produced a shift in the type of diagnostic categories used in the hospital, as Clouston replaced the existing, somewhat eclectic, system based on Skae's aetiological classification with a more uniform and standardised one. Following Clouston's own logic, then, the statistical increase in patients diagnosed with melancholia was at least in part the result of different diagnostic practices. While key symptoms were often initially noted on the patient's medical certificate, a formal diagnosis was assigned by an asylum physician once the patient had been admitted. To recap briefly from Chapter 5, when a person was to be admitted into the asylum they would first be examined by two physicians[7] who would each sign a medical certificate including descriptions of the 'facts indicating insanity' in the person to be certified. This would include any 'symptoms', such as 'mental depression', 'excitement', 'incoherence', 'delusions', 'poor memory', and so on. Accompanying the medical certificates would be a reception order signed by whoever was having the patient committed—usually a relative, friend, guardian, or poorhouse official. This person would have to note on the form whether the suspected lunatic was 'epileptic', 'suicidal', or 'dangerous to others'. When the patient arrived in the asylum, the information about their state of mind would be transferred to the casebook, and added to this would be various details about the lunatic's mental and physical state upon admission. Finally, within a few days, a diagnosis would be entered based upon the information given.

These acts had to take place before a person was counted as 'melancholic' in asylum statistics, and in this process various phenomena were observed in light of those already noted. A noteworthy feature of the vast number of melancholics admitted into Morningside during Clouston's reign was the widely diverse range of human activities and expressions that were merged under the melancholia banner and read as signs of mental depression and suicidality. This is particularly striking when one considers that during the period considered here—from the mid-1870s until the turn of the twentieth century—melancholia was in published material, including the several editions of Clouston's textbook, described in remarkably standardised language with a relatively homogenous range of symptoms. As melancholia was solidified as an independent diagnosis with a precise symptom picture in the last quarter of the century, the contrast between the casebook and the textbook was significant. Typical 'textbook' cases were at times noted on the pages of casebooks—patients described as suffering from a profound depression, suicidal tendencies, and delusions of guilt and wrongdoing. But just as common were cases marked by difference and individuality who corresponded poorly to the formally defined criteria of the diagnosis. Following from this, it should also be noted that one of the symptoms repeatedly emphasised by Clouston as a defining feature of melancholia—'mental pain'—was virtually absent as a descriptive term in Morningside's patient records.

A comparison between asylum case records and published literature illustrates the complex procedures and negotiations that took place when Victorian physicians attempted to define, delineate, and diagnose mental disease. It also sheds further light on one particular symptom of melancholia that was a key focus of Chapter 5: suicidal tendencies. Clouston and his peers pointed to the annual statistical reports of their institution as evidence for the growing incidence of suicidality among the insane, and in particular the overwhelming prevalence of suicidal behaviour in melancholia. While each asylum necessarily had many of its own characteristics in this period, a number of clinical and administrative features were equally shared. In large part this was a result of attempts by the Lunacy Commission to standardise practices, but the increasing move towards professional association and a sharp rise in the number of asylum physicians who published books and articles based on their clinical observations also played a significant part in facilitating an increasingly homogenous professional environment. The Scottish Board of Commissioners allowed greater managerial freedom for its asylum superintendents than did the English Lunacy Commission; however, in the case of Morningside this had the effect of bringing this institution closer to the standard practices advocated by the English Commissioners. Clouston was a prominent figure in the emerging profession of psychological medicine, he was a moderniser and a prolific publisher, inspired by the latest advances in physiological psychology and internal medicine. The Royal Edinburgh Asylum serves as a fitting space within which to investigate the role of clinical and administrative practices in the production of melancholia as an increasingly standardised diagnosis. Its records serve as the primary case study of this chapter, alongside records from Bethlem (London), Brookwood (Surrey), and Ticehurst (Sussex). As the records of these institutions show, significant intellectual work was required in order to forge a demonstrable correspondence between what was observed on asylum wards and what was presented in textbooks and journal articles.

A Note on Asylum Records

To describe the existing scholarly literature on the Victorian asylum as extensive is an understatement. Volumes have been written about virtually every aspect of what went on inside the walls of these institutions as well as about their place within wider social structures.[8] Andrew Scull has suggested that any 'grand' or general claims about insanity can 'be adequately tested, refined, and extended only on the basis of careful case studies of a range of asylums: studies which grasp the relationship of local developments to the broader national picture, but which simultaneously exploit the opportunity offered by the possibility of a more intensive examination of the history of an individual asylum'.[9] Elsewhere, Scull has lamented what he sees as historiography of psychiatry and of the asylum largely divided along disciplinary lines, with the 'broader scholarly perspective' having chiefly fallen within the purview of sociology while historians have tended to focus 'on the micro-politics of insanity'.[10]

It has certainly been the case that many historians of the asylum have tended to favour the local; what such studies search for, perhaps, is 'not generalizable laws, but contextualised meanings of madness'.[11] Scholars have made extensive use of the staggering wealth of paperwork left behind by the large pauper asylums produced by Victorian bureaucracy. From oversized casebooks, to pecuniary records, to diet tables, building plans, and both private and official correspondence, these documents with their faint odour of disinfectant and mould have allowed historians to speak about the place of the asylum in Victorian society, and the place of the patient in the asylum. Analyses of admissions records offer data on gender, class, religious persuasion, and, of course, diagnoses. Casebooks recount a plethora of 'delusions', vast amounts of drugs administered, methods of force-feeding, and recoveries, as well as conflicts, frustrations, deaths, and autopsies. Melling and Forsythe's study of the Devon county asylums briefly referred to in the Introduction sought to do what Scull prescribed—situate the local in a broader context.[12] Other narrators have used asylum records to trace changing practices in a specific context,[13] or to draw attention to previously obscured factors in admission and diagnosis, subjecting asylum records to scrutiny which seeks to problematise the data on offer rather than take the recorded figures for granted.[14]

Such rich histories have demystified the Victorian asylum for contemporary readers, and highlight the central role these institutions played in the foundation of psychiatry as a modern discipline and branch of medicine. Crucially, asylums were key to the development of diagnostic practices and categories. Anne Goldberg suggests that medical diagnoses such as melancholia 'present solely the voice of the physician, and an abstract voice at that. They tell us something (but not much) of medical practices at the time, but next to nothing about the patient'.[15] It is certainly doubtful whether much can be learnt about the patients behind the medical labels from studying asylum records, but the development of diagnostic categories was closely intertwined with medical practices in a mutually productive relationship. Diagnostic literature informed clinical practices, and vice versa, as is still the case today. It follows that a comprehensive understanding of either of these necessitates an interrogation of their relationship. While physicians presented their nosologies and noteworthy case studies in textbooks and journals, published material gives only a partial picture of the process whereby diagnostic categories were produced, refined, and standardised.

Three of the institutions whose records are drawn upon in this chapter have been the focus of rich historical studies that, taken together, illustrate the complex relationship between local practices, central directives, and theoretical works on psychopathology.[16] This chapter does not, however, go into detail about the individual asylums, about life inside their walls or the people who resided or worked there. The aim in this chapter is not to say something meaningful about the people who went into the asylum and became patients, or the family members or workhouse officials who had them committed, or the physicians who diagnosed them. The concern here is with the production of psychiatric knowledge about people. As noted in the Introduction, asylum records are here read as textual sources; as a crucial component of the intellectual work that produced melancholia as a biomedical mental disease with an increasingly standardised symptomatology. While the previous chapters considered the various theoretical and administrative frameworks that were central to this process, the present chapter maps how the melancholia diagnosis was shaped as it travelled back and forth between the textbook and the casebook.

THOMAS CLOUSTON
AND THE MODERNISATION OF MORNINGSIDE

The Edinburgh Royal Asylum at Morningside offers a fitting space for interrogating the relationship between asylum case notes and published literature in the late nineteenth century. The hospital's superintendent, Thomas Clouston, was one of the period's most prolific and influential writers on mental disease, and Morningside was at the time one of the largest institutions for the insane in Britain. It admitted both pauper and private patients (at various rates), and a significant portion of its patients were admitted from across the border, from as far away as Newcastle. Morningside's medical records and the publications of its staff are the focal point of this chapter, situated in the wider context of published literature on melancholia at the turn of the century, and contrasted with case notes from three other asylums.

English lunacy law and administration were briefly outlined in Chapter 5. In Scotland, legal reform of the asylum system came more than a decade after the Lunacy Acts were passed for England and Wales. Following reports of ill-treatment and neglect, a Royal Commission was appointed in 1855 to investigate the care of lunatics in Scotland's asylums and licensed houses. The Commission concluded that abuse was widespread and drastic reform was required.[17] With the Lunacy (Scotland) Act passed in 1857, a centralised system similar to the English one was created, to be overseen by a Board of Commissioners who were tasked to inspect Scottish asylum on an annual basis and ensure that standards of management, care, and treatment were upheld.[18] Physicians were to submit yearly reports on the state of their institutions, including statistical tables pertaining to the asylum population. By the 1860s the British lunacy bureaucracy was largely complete, with institutions across England, Scotland, and Wales operating under similar centralised systems and regularly producing a wealth of statistical data about the patients residing within their walls. The Scottish Lunacy Act contained much the same provisions as the two British Acts, but a number of practical differences existed. For instance, Scottish asylums were more likely to house both private and pauper patients, and in some cases did not deploy these two distinct categories. There were beds available for people of various means, and Clouston took pride in Morningside's ability to provide high-quality care for patients of modest middle-class backgrounds who would not qualify for subsidised treatment but who would not be able to pay the same rate as private patients from the higher social strata.[19] Another significant, and related, difference was that two medical certificates were required for both private and pauper patients. In addition a 'petition' (later reception order) needed to be signed, usually by a relative or poor law official. All documentation would be submitted to the Sheriff who would then decide whether or not the person should be sent to the asylum.[20]

Clouston took over the running of the Morningside Asylum near Edinburgh upon the death of its former superintendent, David Skae, in 1873. Clouston had received his medical training at Edinburgh, where he had studied under Thomas Laycock among others. He went on to train under Skae immediately after obtaining his medical degree, after which he was offered the role of medical superintendent at Cumberland and Westmorland Asylum in Carlisle where he remained for a decade. Clouston was the definition of a rising star among his peers—by the time he took charge of Morningside he had already been co-editor (with Maudsley) of the *Journal of Mental Science* for a year, and had published a number of articles on mental disease. He would go on to become one of the most prolific writers of his peer group, and remained the head of Morningside until well into the first decade of the next century.[21]

Clouston was firmly wedded to a modern scientific approach to mental disease, and was inspired by the work of physiologists such as Carpenter and Laycock. The latter had assumed the chair of the practice of medicine and clinical medicine at Edinburgh University in 1855, and also gave the university's lectures on mental diseases.[22] When Clouston took over as head of Edinburgh's major asylum the two men made a 'private arrangement' to combine their theoretical and practical knowledge of mental disease. In a lecture delivered at the university three years after Laycock's death, Clouston praised his friend and mentor for his leading contributions in the field of 'cerebral physiology and pathology'.[23] He subsequently filled Laycock's role as a lecturer in mental diseases, allowing him to combine his clinical experience with the theoretical teaching of psychological medicine. Clouston's early lectures at Edinburgh formed the foundation for his first textbook, *Clinical Lectures on Mental Diseases* (1883).

Clouston's ascent to the position of superintendent at the Royal Edinburgh Asylum was immediately noticeable in the practice of taking patient notes. Mid-way through 1873, the system of classification used at Morningside was transformed rather abruptly, with the result that it conformed more closely to the standard nosology recommended by the English Lunacy Commission. As discussed in Chapter 5, in England and Wales the Lunacy Commission strongly encouraged nosological unity across asylums, urging physicians to adopt its recommended system of classification, and providing asylums with pre-printed forms for recording signs and symptoms of mental disease. However, the Scottish Board of Commissioners took a different approach, allowing physicians to choose the system they found most useful. George Robertson, Clouston's successor at Morningside, praised this decision in a 1920 historical review of the Scottish lunacy system, suggesting that it encouraged innovation and prevented stagnation.[24] In the case of Edinburgh, it meant that the asylum was reformed along modern scientific lines when Clouston was appointed to run it, as he chose to steer Morningside largely along the lines favoured by the Lunacy Commission across the border.

The freedom awarded to Scottish asylum physicians in the management of their institutions meant that Skae had been able to deploy a wholly individual nosology. He had developed his own system of classification based on the presumed causes of mental disease rather than observable symptoms, divided into twenty-five categories (and two subcategories), such as 'phthisical insanity', 'post-connubial insanity', 'ovarian insanity', 'asthenic insanity', and 'traumatic insanity'.[25] Under Skae's management, his own system was used in conjunction with more widely accepted categories such as melancholia, mania, monomania, moral insanity, and dementia, so that some patients received a diagnosis from Skae's system, and some received one of the more common labels. When Clouston took over in the summer of 1873, the more standard categories were immediately deployed across the board. From this point onwards, the majority of patients arriving at Morningside were diagnosed with mania, melancholia, general paralysis, or dementia, with the odd case of monomania, moral insanity, and imbecility. Skae's system was initially preserved as a secondary diagnostic tool in addition to the primary diagnosis, but gradually fell out of use.

As well as enforcing a standardised system of classification, in 1874 Clouston introduced casebooks with pre-printed headings. The old casebooks used under Skae had consisted of numbered blank pages, whereas the new ones came with several pre-printed sections with various subheadings, including basic information such as age, sex, religion, and occupation. When a patient was admitted to Morningside, the attending physician was now required to state whether there was a 'hereditary history of insanity', what the patient's 'first' and 'recent' 'mental' and 'physical' symptoms were, whether they harboured any 'morbid habits or propensities', and whether the patient was 'suicidal' or 'dangerous'. Following these sections, the 'facts indicating insanity' given in the two medical certificates was to be entered. The second page of a new case was devoted solely to the patient's 'state on admission', requiring the attending physician to note any signs of 'exaltation', 'depression', 'excitement', or 'enfeeblement', whether the patient was 'coherent', had a reasonable 'memory', and whether they exhibited any 'delusions'. At the bottom of the page, after a long list of bodily functions to be assessed, a diagnosis was to be entered. This was followed by a separate heading asking for a second diagnosis according to 'Skae's classification'; this space was, however, for the most part left blank.

The information entered on the first two pages of each new patient's records constituted the foundational data for the statistical report compiled by Clouston and submitted to the Board of Commissioners on a yearly basis. He composed Morningside's annual reports with impressive breadth and detail, and included his own analytical discussions of the statistics presented therein.[26] Clouston's meticulousness and emphasis on rigorous standards and consistency in recording practices were made explicit in his first report to the Board of Commissioners at the end of 1873:

> On the admission of every patient, as complete a medical history of the causes of his disease, and his previous symptoms, as can be obtained from the person who accompanied him from the Asylum, is taken down by one of the Assistant Physicians, who then examines carefully into the symptoms present, and afterwards keeps a record of the changes that take place. This procedure I regard as of the utmost importance to the patient in every way, if done thoroughly and systematically. I have brought into use for the purpose printed forms with suitable headings, so that nothing may be omitted in any case.[27]

These 'printed forms', then, ensured that certain types of information were noted in every case. The presence of pre-printed headings also meant that it was possible to note various aspects of the patient's condition with a simple 'yes' or 'no', or with other brief affirmative or negative responses. Thus, the attending physician only had to give a single word answer to questions of whether the patient was 'suicidal' or exhibited signs of 'depression'. The forms left the choice of diagnosis open-ended;

thus, while Skae's nosology was no longer used as a source of primary diagnoses, the statistical tables of diagnostic categories would change subtly from one year to the next. Certain types of mental disease featured in every annual report, specifically mania, melancholia, general paralysis, and dementia, with the first two being further divided into a number of subcategories. In the first report under Clouston, we find in addition twelve cases of 'moral insanity' and one case of 'monomania' among the new admissions of that year. As noted above, the following year Clouston remarked upon a notable increase in the number of melancholic patients admitted, suggesting that this development was 'very striking, and of great interest', emphasising the importance of vigilance in the face of the persistent suicidal tendencies of such patients.[28]

For the year 1874, 67 patients were reported to be 'suicidal', of whom 38 were diagnosed with some form of melancholia. In a detailed analysis of the annual reports of Morningside, Allan Beveridge suggests that Clouston recognised eight subtypes of melancholia: 'simple; hypochrondriacal; delusional; excited; restive; epileptiform; organic; and suicidal and homicidal'.[29] The categories Beveridge lists are drawn from Clouston's *Clinical Lectures on Mental Diseases*. However, the categories presented in the book took some time to refine. In 1874 we meet with some additional subtypes of melancholia which appear to bear the traces of Skae's classification, such as 'traumatic', 'puerperal', 'senile', and 'melancholia of lactation'.[30] Between 1873 and 1900 melancholia was gradually and subtly standardised in Clouston's report to the Board of Commissioners. Certain subcategories disappeared and others became more common. At the same time, the 'very striking' proportion of melancholic cases which prompted Clouston's comments in 1874 would from thereon become the norm; indeed the most striking thing about these figures is perhaps that while melancholia continued to be diagnosed with growing frequency, Clouston never again remarked upon this development.

A 'Typical' Case of Melancholia

The description of melancholia offered by Clouston in *Clinical Lectures* was clear and precise: it was an illness characterised by 'emotional depression' and 'mental pain', often leading to 'uncontrollable impulses towards suicide', and sometimes accompanied by a 'loss of self-control' or 'delusions', a lack of interest in a capacity for most common activities, and with slowed bodily functions. Like Griesinger, Clouston placed melancholia under the banner 'states of mental depression', which he also referred to as 'psychalgia', fusing to an extent the symptoms of depression and mental pain in the same way Griesinger had done. Moreover, like the German psychiatrist had also done some decades earlier, Clouston emphasised that these states were 'of all forms of mental diseases those that are nearest mental health'. Following from this, he highlighted mental pain as a particularly interesting symptom, as this was a sensation also experienced by healthy people:

> To be able to feel pain implies an encephalic tissue for the purpose. To be very sensitive to pain implies that the tissue is acutely receptive of impressions. So with mental pain there can be no doubt that the healthy physiological condition of the encephalic tissue in the brain convolutions through which ordinary or mental pain is felt is one between extreme callousness to impressions and extreme sensitiveness. A man in robust health, well exercised, does not feel pain nearly so acutely, and bears it better than when he is weak and run down. Those principles apply equally to the feeling and bearing of mental pain. To experience emotion at all – *to feel* – implies an encephalic structure for this purpose. The most casual study of the affective capacity in humans show us that it differs enormously in different persons.[31]

Added to a brain's level of sensitivity was its inhibitory power—its capacity for enduring pain. These two aspects of the cerebral physiology of pain together held the key to understanding the potential ability for mental pain to become pathological: 'when a brain is sensitive, and has little inhibitory power, this combination is a source of weakness and of disease'.[32] Such mental pain was a defining feature of melancholia, a diseased state that could be easily distinguished from 'a mere feeling of melancholy' since a 'typical case of melancholia [...] runs a somewhat definite course, like a fever, and has often all the characters of an acute disease'.[33] Clouston suggested that melancholia was by far the easiest form of mental disease to examine and diagnose, as patients were generally aware of their suffering and able to communicate it and answer questions. At the commencement of an examination, he suggested, the melancholia patient 'will tell you in the first place very likely that he is unhappy, and feels mental pain and depression'. The 'unsoundness of mind' would manifest when asking patients for the cause of this suffering, as they would almost invariably 'assign as a cause of their misery what is not its cause at all'.[34] However, as will be seen below, there was no mention in the Morningside casebooks of patients themselves using the words 'depression' and 'mental pain' to express their emotional state.

Any student consulting Clouston's textbook would be furnished with clear instructions for how to identify melancholia: look for the expression, in words and countenance, of mental pain and depression, a general lack of interest, and be attentive to any signs of suicidal intent. Moreover, patients would most likely attribute their suffering to an illusionary cause, such as having committed a terrible sin. Cases of simple melancholia, by far the most common, would rarely be sent to the asylum as they could be treated at home, but were nonetheless important to identify and diagnose to prevent deterioration of the condition. In these cases, 'the affective depression or pain is far more marked than the intellectual and volitional aberrations'.[35] Clouston presented a 'typical' case of this form of the disease, a gentleman in his sixties whose emotional health had begun to decline following 'a big piece of intellectual work'. He became tired, depressed, lost interest in his usual duties, and was unable to feel the same affection for his wife and children as he had previously done. Confused by these feelings, he believed that they 'must be a judgement on him for some sin'. With time his mental suffering grew more severe, his delusions of guilt more profound, and his whole constitution became affected. Upon examining the patient, Clouston recommended rest, a journey to the sea, and an 'easily digested but fattening diet'.[36]

Clouston supplemented this case with a line of similar 'typical' cases of simple melancholia, followed by the closely related hypochondriacal variety, before proceeding to the more profound, 'delusional' melancholia. Contrary to Maudsley, Clouston found the suicidal propensity to be more common in this than in the simple form, as the mental suffering was usually more severe. In these forms of delusional melancholia, Clouston argued, many patients experienced real or imagined abdominal discomfort, often resulting in a refusal of food, which in the most critical cases could only be resolved through force-feeding with the stomach pump. He recounted a number of such typical cases, characterised by profound depression of mind, delusions both of a religious and a hypochondriacal nature (pertaining to the gastric region), persistent suicidal tendencies, and a refusal of food leading the patients to be forcefed. With some variations, the similarities with Moses B., the typical case of suicidal melancholia met with at the start of this chapter, are striking.[37]

.

However, Clouston also noted a type of melancholia—Excited (Motor) Melancholia—that exhibited some more uncommon, markedly excited, features, resulting from 'epileptiform attacks'. Such involuntary reactions were attributed to the relationship referred to above between the brain's sensitivity and its inhibitory power, whereby a combination of an intense response to stimuli and a lack of cerebral inhibition resulted in violent involuntary motor reactions. This type of melancholia was particularly common in 'the Celtic race' and in women in general, Clouston argued, illustrated by the 'wailing and weeping, the gesticulations and motor grief of an Irish woman', reactions that were 'usually out of all proportion to the mental pain'. Recounting a typical case of this form of the disease, Clouston described the familiar symptoms of melancholia, suggesting that the female patient 'attempted suicide', was upon admission 'greatly depressed', and 'confessed to feeling exceedingly miserable'. After a few days in the asylum her depression grew deeper, and she 'thought she was to be killed, and that everything was going wrong with her; did not take her food well; attempted to drown herself by jumping into the asylum shallow curling pond'. The excited motor features were exhibited as an expression of her despair: 'She wrings her hands; sways backwards and forwards, contorting her body; rushes about from place to place, and cannot settle for a minute'.[38] Again the reader was presented with a typical case featuring all the usual symptoms of melancholia, but with the added aspect of involuntary motor action arising from, and reflecting, the particular quality of this mental disturbance.

In a lecture delivered to the asylum staff a few years later, in 1887, Clouston reiterated his earlier definition of melancholia as predominantly characterised by mental pain, suggesting that '[l]ove of life is a natural instinct, but when the brain is diseased, as in Melancholia, the love of life is lost. Melancholia is the least marked kind of insanity; every kind of insanity begins with it as the first symptom. The feelings, intellect, &c., are all disturbed, and the chief symptom is mental pain'.[39] Like many of his peers, Clouston held this mental pain to be a significant cause of the suicidal propensity in melancholia. He emphasised that 'while no tendency to suicide exists at all in many melancholics', it should nonetheless always be carefully watched out for since 'it does exist in some form or other, in wish, intention, or act, in four out of every five of all the cases'.[40] Nevertheless, Clouston found it useful to note a separate category of 'suicidal melancholia' closely related to a less common 'homicidal' type. This type of the disease was, he argued, 'the most striking and most important'. In a remark similar to those made by Maudsley and Mercier a few years later,[41] Clouston perceived suicidality as a complete reversal of the evolutionary drive for self-preservation:

> When the love of life, that primary and strongest instinct, not only in man, but in all the animal kingdom, through which continuous acts of self-preservation of the individual life of every living thing take place, when that is lost, and not only lost but reversed, so that a man craves to die as strongly as he ever craved to live, we have then the greatest change in the instinctive and affective faculties of man that is possible, and have reached the acme of all states of mental depression.[42]

However, like Maudsley and Mercier, Clouston went on to note that this utter reversal of the natural instinct could, paradoxically, at the same time constitute a natural, indeed sane reaction when occurring as a response to profound mental pain. 'The determination to commit suicide is in some cases one come to in the calmest and most reasonable way', he suggested, and in such instances was 'nearest in character to the suicides among sane persons'. However, in a large number of cases of melancholia, the suicidal tendency was equally bound up with severe and frightening delusions arising from mental pain and depression, most often delusions of guilt tied to the belief that the patient had committed a great sin against God and her or his family and friends, and therefore did not deserve to live. The suicidal tendency in melancholia was thus a feature of the disease that much preoccupied Clouston, not just from the point of view of patient safety, but also as a riddle in the philosophy and biology of life. This interest in suicidality was much in evidence both in his annual reports to the Board of Commissioners, and in the way patients' symptoms were assessed and noted in the Morningside casebooks. Indeed, most of these distinctions between different types of melancholia listed in Clouston's published work and annual reports were not made in the Morningside casebooks, with the exception of suicidality. The single diagnosis would be entered, and often followed by an abbreviated reference to suicidal tendencies in brackets. The notes made as to a patient's suicidality would be tallied up at the end of the year and entered into neat columns listing the total number of 'suicidal' patients, which diagnoses were represented among them, and how many had 'meditated' or 'attempted' suicide. Through these different acts of recording, counting, summarising, and listing, then, a vast range of activities and expressions communicated and observed on the wards created two categories that featured in reports and published literature, not just in Edinburgh, but across Britain—the 'typical' case of melancholia, and the 'suicidal' patient. A closer look at asylum records reveals that both categories suggested simplicity and coherence that was not mirrored in the myriad of symptoms displayed by asylum patients who received these labels.

Typical and Untypical Cases: Melancholia from the Textbook to the Asylum Ward

In the final decades of the century, an increasing number of asylums introduced casebooks with pre-printed sections for recording patient history, symptoms, and diagnosis. This formed part of, and helped facilitate, a broad shift in record taking from longer, discursive descriptions of patients' mental states to briefer statements and descriptive keywords. Two concerns in particular drove this development. On the one hand, the requirement to provide uniform and comparable statistical data on patient populations and diagnostics produced a need for standardised recording practices. On the other hand, these changes to how patient data was recorded were also facilitated by time constraints at a time when asylums and their populations were rapidly expanding across the country. This shift in the practice of note-taking was mirrored across much of Western medicine in the second half of the nineteenth century; a development that one historian has referred to as a 'new epistemological and aesthetic sensibility, expressed as a narrative preference for what was universal and precise over what was individual and discursive'.[43]

The casebooks at Morningside illustrate this shift. In earlier years, under Skae's management, case notes had been comprehensive, discursive narratives of each patient's history, state of mind, and bodily condition. With the pre-printed casebooks introduced by Clouston in the 1870s, a few key terms were often deemed sufficient. While the amount and format of the information entered varied, sometimes considerably, depending on which physician entered it, the overall trend was towards briefer, more precise descriptions, centring on single words or abbreviated sentences. The trend for briefer language was particularly prominent in the description of symptoms. The act of condensing information was notable in the 'facts indicating insanity' transferred from the medical certificates to the casebook, where the explanations given by the two certifying physicians were increasingly summarised into a few keywords. In the case of

Isabella K., a rather typical case of melancholia admitted in the summer of 1893, the first of the medical certificates accompanying her to the asylum suggested that the patient 'talks incoherently and has delusions that she has ceased to live. She does not know the year nor the day of week. Has great depression. Melancholia'. Added to this were the 'facts' told by her husband, who was said to confirm this assessment of her mental state, adding that 'she has been ill for about ten days and has lost her memory'. The second medical certificate claimed Isabella K. to be 'very depressed and melancholic, says that she is lost and that her maker has devised a punishment for her disobedience to his will to be burning in Hell', and that 'her husband states that for ten days she has been very depressed, forgetting everything'.[44]

On the first page of her casebook entry, this already brief information about the patient's state of mind was entered under the heading 'Facts of Medical Certificates' simply as 'Looks depressed. Delusions. Bad memory'. She was further noted as 'suicidal' and where the physician was required by the pre-printed headings to note the presence or absence of 'depression', the answer given was 'Considerable. Looks unhappy'. It was not stated in what her suicidal tendency consisted, except in the single word 'threatened'.[45] Overall the format of casebook entries under Clouston's management produced these kinds of brief, concise descriptions where patients' mental states were described as key symptoms, such as 'depression', 'delusions of a religious nature', and so on. This practice had the effect of creating an increasingly homogenous set of symptoms, as the more personalised narratives of individual patients were gradually erased. We meet, then, with a large number of 'typical' cases of melancholia, similar to that of Isabella K. above, and of Moses B., the young suicidal doctor whose case was discussed at the start of this chapter.

One such typical case, fifty-five-year-old Dorothy D. admitted in 1876, was described in the following terms: 'Became depressed and melancholy', 'Refused Food', 'Has attempted suicide several times; by knife, hanging, &c. and wishes to drown herself'. 'Is very depressed in spirits, and imputes blame to herself for all sorts of imaginary sins'. Her state of mind upon admission was noted as 'Depression great – shown by her conversation and the expression of her countenance; says that she has ruined her husband and family, that she injures and destroys everything near her, that she has done great wrong, &c'. Such typical cases of melancholia abounded; individuals who came into the asylum and ticked most of the boxes for common forms of melancholia: mental depression, suicidal tendencies, and religious delusions, but who were generally clear-headed enough to answer questions and express how they felt. Pauline N., admitted in the same year as Dorothy, was an equally typical melancholic, her most prominent mental symptoms noted as 'depression and suicidal tendency', and according to both of the certifying physicians believed herself to be 'under a curse from her birth', due to which she had 'ruined her family'. Her state upon admission to Morningside was recounted as characterised by 'great depression shown by her depressed self-absorbed expression and demeanour'. Twenty-five-year-old Margaret L. was an equally typical case, having become 'depressed' as a result of 'anxiety' relating to her work. An assistant in her grain merchant father's business, the exciting cause of her melancholia was believed to be her sister's recent move to America, 'throwing the whole charge of business on her'. Described as 'suicidal', one of the physicians certifying her lunacy stated that she had declared 'that she wished to destroy herself, that she may not be a burden to her parents', adding that according to her father 'she took poison on Thursday, and this morning she threw herself over the window from a height of three flats'. When first examined upon her arrival at the asylum, her mental state was given as one of 'considerable depression, shown by her expression, and by her conversation. She says she wishes to destroy herself, as she is the cause of ruin to her father'.[46] Similarly, Alexander H., admitted in 1877, was described as 'depressed' and 'low in spirits' and having 'attempted suicide by taking laudanum'. The attending physician at Morningside assessed his mental condition as 'Depression great, shown by his expression, manner, and conversation, and by the nature of his delusions. Says that he feels very dull and that he is lost forever'.[47]

Apparently absent from these and many more 'typical' cases were, however, any account by the patients themselves of suffering from 'depression', or from 'mental pain'. Indeed, the latter did not feature as a symptom in the Morningside casebooks at all. What these casebooks reveal, then, is the process, today standard practice in psychiatric diagnostics, of translating patients' various complaints, verbal and non-verbal expressions, past and present acts, and reported medical history into certain symptom terms—universally applicable keywords that serve to merge together the chaos of human activity into simplified medical labels. With a rapidly growing asylum population, and a perceived need for a more unified language between medical psychologists, the increased use of unifying keywords such as depression and mental pain served important practical uses for late Victorian asylum physicians. It enabled swifter description and recording of a patient's mental state, as well as facilitating the assembly of statistical tables over diagnoses and symptoms. It also aided the dissemination and publication of cases within the wider peer community by producing a nomenclature that was accessible and comprehensible to anyone with professional knowledge in the field of mental disease. When one physician published an article about a particularly interesting or representative case, such as that of Moses B., the use of terms such as 'suicidal' and 'depressed' would immediately make the patient's state of mind appear familiar to the professional reader.

However, while the act of merging an endless range of human activities into simplified key terms made descriptions of symptoms and diagnoses of disease more precise, it equally served to flatten out a highly uneven field of psychological phenomena. The use of singular keywords precluded the need for more detailed narrative descriptions of individual experiences—one of its greatest benefits to the busy physician, but equally an act that had the effect of producing new information about people. As noted above, in the decades following Clouston's ascendancy to the position of superintendent at Morningside, the casebook descriptions grew increasingly brief and concise, and included less and less variation in the terminology used to note the patients' mental states. One of the shifts that took place with the introduction of pre-printed headings was a decline in reasons given for assigning a particular symptom. In other words, descriptions became decidedly *un*-descriptive. This was particularly the case with 'depression', one of the key features that required noting as part of a new patient's state upon admission. In the case of Dorothy D. referred to above, her 'depression' was observed in 'her conversation and the expression of her countenance'. Similarly, Janet G.'s 'depression' was described as 'Great, looks very unhappy, cries',[48] Alexander Duffle's depression was noted as 'Great. Expression is one of misery and he is continually crying',[49] Jane Ann C.'s depression was 'exhibited in manner, appearance, and communication', Isabella Hutton's depression was 'marked, exhibited in appearance and conversation',[50] Robert G.'s depression was 'Considerable. Looks unhappy and confused, and cried while being examined',[51] and Catherine G.'s depression was simply 'present in her expression'.[52]

Contrary to Clouston's remark in his textbooks, patients did not themselves appear to express a feeling of being 'depressed'. As noted above, depression, mental pain, and suicidal tendencies were descriptive terms deployed by physicians as identifiable symptoms, keywords to describe a certain state of mind that was perceived as widespread among asylum patients, but which said little about what those patients themselves expressed about their emotional states. David Walker and Anita O'Connell have noted the homogenising function of depression as a single descriptive term for a range of emotional states associated with low mood, remarking that it 'not only replaced a wider vocabulary for a variety of experiences', but that it 'also flattened out the individuality' of those experiences.[53] Only fragments of individual expressions can be glimpsed in the brief narratives given of patient interviews, where a vast range of thoughts and feelings were described. John W., whose depression was stated as 'marked', expressed according to the attending physician a fear 'that the persons around him are wishing to injure him, and is constantly crying out "You won't kill me, you won't kill me"',[54] whereas Elizabeth F. told the medical officer examining her that she believed herself to have been poisoned as a result of 'some sin she committed in her youth', and that she was now eternally lost.[55] Isabelle H. expressed that 'she is not human, that she has no feelings and that she would like to die',[56] and Peter S. claimed that 'the devil is after him and that people are suspicious of him'. Other patients said very little at all, appearing reluctant and unable to answer any questions put to them. Robert M., a pauper patient admitted in 1887, would 'not answer any questions or answers them incoherently, constantly repeats the same words, as "the man", "the man"',[57] while Isaac W. was described as 'taciturn and disinclined to answer questions',[58] and Isabella M. 'Refuses to answer all direct questions' and displayed a 'vacant look'.[59]

This conflation of different expressions under the label depression was equally reflected in the casebooks of other British asylums in this period, such as Surrey Country Asylum at Brookwood, which was run by Thomas Brushfield. The casebooks at Brookwood tell a similar story to those of Morningside, and contain a large number of typical and untypical cases of melancholia. Frances H., a 38-year-old nurse admitted into Brookwood in 1879 and diagnosed with melancholia was recorded as suicidal and suffering from 'depression of spirits without apparent cause', which manifested in that she 'does not know what she shall do and feels suicidal' and 'is not regular'.[60] Julia P., a young woman admitted into the same asylum the previous year was also recorded as depressed and suicidal with 'religious delusions'. The evidence for her mental state consisted in that she 'said the Devil was constantly after her and that she feels as if she must kill herself'.[61] Similarly, William W., who was brought to Brookwood from Lambeth workhouse in 1871, was described as depressed, 'very' suicidal, and having 'delusional views of religion', which led him to believe that 'there is no time for him left to repent and that his sins have been so great'.[62] Like Morningside, Brookwood had recently introduced casebooks with pre-printed sections, which made it easier for attending physicians to record mental symptoms, in particular the presence of suicidal tendencies, where a simple yes or no was sufficient. Suicidality appeared with high frequency in conjunction with the melancholia diagnosis, which was reflected in the asylum's annual statistical reports. Depression on the other hand was not included in the pre-printed section (unlike at Morningside), but it was nevertheless by far the most frequently noted mental symptom in melancholic patients alongside suicidal tendencies.

A similar picture emerges from the casebooks of Ticehurst, a private licensed facility in Sussex run by the Newingtons, a family of physicians, and where Henry Maudsley occasionally consulted. While private institutions were subject to inspection, they were not under the same administrative pressure as county asylums with regard to data collection. However, recording practices generally mirrored those of public institutions. By the mid-1870s, pre-printed casebooks were also in use at Ticehurst, which asked among other things whether the patient admitted was suicidal. Depression equally appeared as the most common mental symptom of melancholia, such as in 44-year-old John S., whose 'depression of spirits' was noted as 'great' and evidenced by 'constantly thinking & troubling about his business & money' and that 'he is unable to fix his attention on anything & that he said last night "you don't know what I am going to do"'. This statement by the patient appears to be the primary reason for suspecting him to harbour suicidal tendencies, alongside a 'refusal of food and medicine'. 42-year-old Caroline Ann W., admitted three years later and diagnosed with melancholia, was equally described as suffering from 'mental depression' and recorded as suicidal. She was reported as stating that 'she was the devil and not fit to live' and that she 'took poison & attempted to destroy herself'. Alongside such 'typical' cases of melancholia with what was at the time familiar signs of 'depression', can be found others such Eliza B., a young woman admitted in the autumn of 1878 and diagnosed as 'melancholic and suicidal', with her mental state described as 'very depressed'. In this case, none of the more common reasons for this term are given, rather the evidence for her depression appears to be that she 'won't eat any meat as she believes she is then responsible for the death of the animals'.

SUICIDAL MELANCHOLICS

As the above cases imply, a number of different expressions and acts suggested to physicians that melancholic patients were depressed, and that they harboured suicidal intentions. In several of his reports to the Board of Commissioners, Clouston remarked upon the growing incidence of suicidal patients under his care, and as suggested above, his annual statistical charts included a table of suicidal tendencies in patients admitted. The total number of suicidal patients was divided into the various forms of mental disease represented, followed by a list of the nature of attempts, where such had been undertaken. Each year the tables indicated that the vast majority of suicidal patients, whether they had 'attempted' or 'meditated', were diagnosed with melancholia. However, when taking a closer look at the patient records that served as the basis for these tables a rather more complex picture emerges.

In his 1887 report to the Commissioners, Clouston emphasised the importance of vigilance in order to prevent 'suicidal' patients from achieving their goal. While deaths by suicide were rare in Morningside (and generally also in other asylums), this year two patients had succeeded in taking their lives, prompting Clouston to reiterate the substantial difficulty for even the trained physician in detecting the presence of suicidal intent in a patient:

> We have no test by which we can infallibly tell the presence or absence of the suicidal impulse – that most subtile, terrible, and sudden of all morbid mental symptoms. It may exist in a man whose mental working is otherwise strong: it may arise in a moment: it may be suggested by any means of taking away life: it may overmaster the strongest resolutions and the best principles; and it may even co-exist in the mind with a horror and loathing of itself.[63]

That year, the number of 'suicidal' patients numbered 79, of whom 61 were melancholic. Of the total number of suicidal patients, 23 were stated to have attempted and the remaining 56 meditated. The types of attempts listed for that year were 'precipitation', 'cut-throat', 'poisoning', 'hanging', 'strangulation', 'drowning', and 'starvation'.[64]

One of these suicidal melancholics was Jane C., who had reportedly become insane following 'domestic bereavement'. She 'grew dull and low spirited', and more recently had become 'very restless and excited and tried to throw herself over the window'. Jane, then, belonged to the category of 'attempted' suicides, and was upon admission described as suffering from 'great depression' and plagued by the delusional belief that 'she has committed unpardonable sins and must go to hell'.[65] She was a typical case of suicidal melancholia, much like the published case of Moses B. Moses had, as noted at the start, been admitted to Morningside after taking 'a poisonous dose of Belladonna', an act that saw him labelled 'suicidal' on his reception order and medical certificates and consequently subject to close monitoring on the asylum ward. According to assistant physician Joseph Brown's article on the case, as well as Moses' casebook entries, his suicide attempts continued once inside the asylum. There, he swallowed several stones, after which he complained of abdominal distress and began to decline his meals. This act of 'refusing his food' was looked upon with severity, as it was undertaken 'evidently with the hope of starving himself'. As a result, the stomach pump was deployed on several occasions. Moses' next suicide attempt reportedly consisted in taking 'an overdose of alcohol', a feat he accomplished after having saved up the small drop of whiskey patients were given with their evening meal each night. Around two weeks after this incident, from which he subsequently recovered, the patient 'snatched' from an attendant a bottle containing 'a solution of guttapercha in chloroform', which he proceeded to drink. Moses became unconscious and only came to several hours later after persistent attempts to revive him. According to Brown, the patient grew steadily stronger over the next few days, but 'continues to refuse his food, and has to be fed with the tube'. The persistence with which Moses apparently pursued his desire to die constituted a demonstrable example of the suicidal tendency in melancholics—so determined did the patient seem in his suicidal convictions that 'his one and only object in life is to destroy it'.[66]

In this one single case, then, a number of acts were presented that were merged under the 'suicidal' banner—swallowing of stones, refusing food, drinking a large quantity of alcohol, and swallowing a poisonous substance. A look at similar 'typical' cases of suicidal melancholia widen the range further. Pauline N. had 'threatened or attempted violence to herself by drowning at the first attack, and during the second by swallowing pins and knocking her head', while Elizabeth F. had 'refused food: saying that she did not want to live' and had according to her husband 'attempted to poison herself'.[67] Isabella M.'s suicidal tendency consisted in 'trying to leave the house in the night, and often refusing her food', John C. had 'twice attempted suicide by cutting his throat', Isabella H. was deemed suicidal because she would walk 'about the streets in a depressed state – found standing on the top balcony to jump over, &c.', and Agnes F.'s suicidality manifested in proclaiming that she was 'desperately miserable and that all she wants is to leave this world'.[68] Robert A., an 'anxious and dejected' widower was labelled suicidal due to having reportedly 'threatened to cut his throat, and has tried to get out of the window', Alexander M. was deemed by one of his certifying physicians to be suicidal after he 'wanted to get a knife', and Jane C. was noted as having 'threatened' suicide after she 'wandered away to the Dean Bridges' but did not jump in the river 'as she says the water was not deep enough'.[69] Alexander D. was described in his case notes as having 'attempted' suicide after having become 'very excited'. While in this state he 'appeared to be suicidal and took hold of a knife. He did not injure himself however'. Robert G. was placed in the category of melancholics who had 'meditated' suicide after he 'asked for a pistol and a rope to destroy himself', as was Alexander B., who 'said that he was tired of life and wished to have done with it, but he has made no actual attempts'.[70] Madeleine M., another case of typical suicidal melancholia, had reportedly been 'refusing food' and 'threw herself before a train', and Catherine G. was described as 'suicidally inclined' after stating 'that she wishes to die'.[71]

In the case of several melancholics who received the label 'suicidal', either in their medical certificate or upon admission, no apparent reason was given for their suicidality; rather, it appeared to be deduced from their general state of mind. Annie V., a 'suicidal' melancholic admitted in the summer of 1898, was noted as harbouring 'melancholic ideas. Thinks there is no food for her children, that she will be had up for ill treatment, &c.', but no other reason for her purported suicidality was given. Similarly, in the case of Elizabeth R. who was admitted the previous winter and reportedly required 'constant watching', the suicidal tendency appeared to be derived from reports that she 'wanders about at night' and 'refuses food'. Refusal of food was equally the reason given for the suspected presence of suicidal intent in Jane Ann C., while in the case of Isabella H. no apparent reason was given beyond the 'usual' symptom of 'depression', deduced from the patient appearing 'dull and melancholy and despondent'. In a number of such cases where the 'suicidal' label came without explanation, such as those of James C. and James W., both admitted in 1888, few symptoms were given beyond the familiar 'depression', 'lowness of spirits', and 'despondency'.[72] In sum, the Morningside casebooks appeared to confirm the belief expressed by Maudsley in 1879, that '[s]uicidal feelings and attempts are common in melancholia, so much so that one suspects their actual or possible existence even when they have not been openly manifested'.[73]

A similar picture emerges from county asylums in England at this time. As noted in Chapter 5, Thomas Brushfield lamented the flawed nature of statistics on suicidality, suggesting that these often included self-injurious acts committed without suicidal intent. In the case of melancholia, however, he took a different approach. As with Morningside, melancholic patients under Brushfield's care were frequently labelled suicidal even in the absence of suicidal acts or openly manifested intent. In the case of John G., a suicidal melancholic admitted to Brookwood shortly after Brushfield took over the running of the asylum in the 1860s, no specific reason was given for considering him to harbour suicidal tendencies, beyond the patient stating that 'he feels very low sometimes but cannot give any reasons for being so'.[74] In patients diagnosed with melancholia, any act or expression that could be construed as having self-injurious intent was likely to be labelled suicidal. Ann F., admitted in 1869, was labelled as suicidal because she 'seemed very much depressed and expressed an intense feeling of melancholy, as if she would do herself an injury'.[75] Ann W., admitted the following year, was also considered to be suicidal, which according to the attending physician manifested in 'persistent refusal of food', while Sarah Elizabeth L. was said to have 'attempted suicide by pressing her fingers slightly round her throat', and for this reason required 'constant watching'.[76]

The previous chapter noted how George Savage equally questioned the validity of statistics on suicidal patients, arguing that many of the suicidal patients under his care were not 'actively' suicidal. By the 1870s, Bethlem was also using pre-printed casebooks, which only required a yes or no as to whether a patient was suicidal. On the pages of Bethlem's casebooks can equally be found a range of acts and expressions merged under the suicidal label, and much as at Morningside and Brookwood, patients' behaviour appeared to be more likely to be labelled suicidal if they were considered to be suffering from melancholia. For instance, Sarah M., admitted in December 1878, when Savage had recently been put in charge, was perceived as suffering from melancholia with typical religious delusions, stating that she had committed 'the unpardonable sin' for which she could 'not be forgiven'. Her suicidality appeared to be attributed to her having 'made several attempts to set fire to the house'. In the case of Alfred N., another suicidal melancholic, his perceived suicide 'attempt' consisted in 'having swallowed...shilling pieces last week, and a penny this morning'. Emma H. was described as labouring under 'extreme depression', believing herself 'to be the most wicked woman in the world'. When she drank 'some liniment', this was seen as an act with suicidal intent.

While a diagnosis of melancholia was likely to result in an assumption that the patient was suicidal, there were at times also more practical reasons for applying both labels to patients. Records of patients transferred to Morningside from St. Cuthbert's, the local poor house, tell a story of difficult to manage patients who were not reported to express any of the usual symptoms of melancholia, including intent to commit suicide, but who were admitted with 'suicidal' against their name and given a melancholia diagnosis. The question of whether to treat lunatics in the poor house infirmary or have them transferred to the asylum was a contentious one; county asylums were generally much better funded, staffed, and equipped, but it was also more costly to care for patients in these institutions, and transfers of pauper lunatics from the workhouse to the county asylum generally needed to be motivated by the inability of staff in the former to care for the person in question.[77] One of the most common ways of doing this was to confirm on the medical certificate and reception order that the lunatic was either 'dangerous' or 'suicidal'. One such case was that of Mary S., admitted from St. Cuthbert's in June of 1888. None of the usual symptoms of melancholia was noted, except that she 'refuses food'. She was described as excited and 'noisy' by a nurse at St. Cuthbert's infirmary, who also reported that Mary 'tries to bite and requires several women to hold her down', and that she was 'requiring restraint by the attendants to prevent her doing mischief and injuring herself in wild attempts to leave the place'.[78] In the case of Robert M., transferred from the same poor house the previous year, commonly described symptoms of melancholia were equally notable by their absence. Little information was given in the case notes as to the reasons for his confinement and for the diagnosis, only that he had 'a depressed expression' and 'is in a constant state of restlessness, always trying to take off his clothes and fumbling with his hands'. His medical certificates and reception order, however, cite the facts indicating insanity recounted by the nurse at St. Cuthbert's, who claimed that Robert was noisy and restless at night, disturbing the other patients in the infirmary, and that he 'works at the bedclothes with his hands and has to be put under restraint'.[79]

As these case studies illustrate, a vast number of different acts and expressions came together to produce the single category 'suicidal', a symptom of melancholia that functioned together with the other most commonly deployed keyword, 'depression'. These two symptoms of mental disease were produced from a chaos of activities, often deduced in part from 'delusions' of guilt and sin—the 'religious delusions' discussed in Chapter 5—or from a patient's 'dull' or 'despondent' demeanour, and from various acts and statements that were interpreted as intent to 'do away with oneself'. The two things most often expressed by melancholic patients themselves, according to their medical notes, were a sense of profound guilt, of having done something terribly wrong, often causing harm, shame, or destruction to one's family, and following from this, a belief that one did not deserve to live and must therefore destroy oneself. No patient was reported as uttering the words 'depression', 'mental pain', or 'suicide'. These are, however, the key features that emerge from the case notes, and from the annual reports to the Board of Commissioners, where the persistent suicidality of Morningside's melancholics was repeatedly emphasised by Clouston as one of the greatest challenges facing the physician in charge of an asylum.

Clouston's statistical tables of the frequency with which 'suicidal propensities' were encountered in the Morningside patients illustrated what had by the 1880s become the standard view among British asylum physicians: of all lunatics melancholics were the most suicidal, and of all suicidal patients the majority were melancholics. Clouston took care to emphasise this feature in his textbook, warning students and fellow practitioners that

> [t]he question of the patient being suicidal should never in any case of melancholia be left unconsidered, and the risk of his becoming suicidal should never in any case be left unprovided for. No tendency to suicide exists at all in many melancholics from beginning to end of their disease, but it does exist in some form or other – in wish, intention, or act – in four out of every five of all the cases, and we can never tell when it is to develop in any patient.[80]

His own statistics supported this claim year after year, yet no self-inflicted death was reported at Morningside until two suicides were recorded in 1879. Overall such cases were rare in Edinburgh and elsewhere, but the expectation of suicide formed a constant preoccupation for asylum physicians as well as for English and Scottish Commissioners in Lunacy. Thus, Clouston echoed the anxiety felt by many of his peers when he remarked that '[t]he fear of it in reference to some one is always more or less present in my mind'.[81]

Nevertheless, Clouston expressed the same kind of scepticism about the reliability of statistics on suicidality as Savage and others had done. In the first (1883) edition of his textbook he subjected the statistics he had accumulated during his time at Morningside to closer scrutiny. As noted above, Clouston's tables of suicidal patients had separated those who had 'attempted' from those who had 'meditated' suicide. Of the last 729 melancholic patients who had been admitted to the institution, the tables indicated that 'four out of five...were more or less suicidal'. However, many of the attempts, he suggested, 'could scarcely be regarded as being very serious'. Moreover, of the total number just below forty per cent came under the heading 'meditated', in other words they 'had spoken of suicide, or given some indication that it had been in their minds'. Clouston concluded that while the suicide risk in melancholia was statistically very high, his experience told him that 'the actual risk of suicide being seriously attempted or accomplished is much less than those figures seem to show'.[82] Nevertheless, the recording practices put in place by Clouston at Morningside contributed to the widely accepted view of a close relationship between melancholia and suicidal tendencies, with consequences for the admission, diagnosis, and care of melancholics in the Victorian period.

Conclusion

The developments mapped in this and the previous chapter have continued to shape perceptions of mood disorders into the twenty-first century, where emotional pain and depression are perceived as closely linked to suicidal thoughts and actions. Closely related to the emergence of suicidality as a category separate from suicide has been the growing focus of psychiatric attention in the late nineteenth and throughout the twentieth century upon 'self-injurious' behaviour. Late Victorian medical psychologists increasingly used the term 'self-mutilation' to describe a range of what they perceived to be non-suicidal acts, such as amputations and castrations; more commonly, however, medical discussion of 'self-mutilating' behaviour referred to 'minor self-mutilations' such as 'skin-picking' and 'hair-plucking'.[83] In present psychiatry, 'non-suicidal self-injury' has become a firmly cemented medical concept[84]; however, the parameters and definitions of what distinguishes suicidal from non-suicidal self-injury have shifted over time as these categories have been reconceptualised in the context of contemporaneous cultural tropes about group and individual behaviours. The history of these psychiatric models of behaviour is beyond the scope of this book, and have been considered elsewhere.[85] However, it is significant to note the varying and multiple medical meanings of different kinds of 'self-injurious' behaviours in the nineteenth century. In sum, 'suicidal' was produced as a multivalent and shifting concept, one which was at the same time remarkably consistent in medico-psychological literature and in administrative and clinical practice for a time. Despite the fact that Victorian physicians themselves acknowledged the ambiguity of the concept and the problems attached to its use in the production of asylum statistics, they nevertheless continued to rely upon this category as a significant diagnostic criterion in the definition of melancholia, and as a useful tool in the determination of a patient's state of mind.

This chapter has traced the relationship between asylum statistics, diagnostic records, and published material to show how melancholia was constituted, modified, reified, and applied as a diagnosis in late Victorian medicine. Melancholia did not exist as a coherent disease entity with clearly distinguished symptoms prior to the practices and the language which sought to identify and classify it. If we want to say something about how psychiatric diagnoses were produced in the nineteenth century (and beyond), we must address the relationship between asylum case notes, which were often messy and inconsistent, and published material where neat psychiatric categories were described together with evidence drawn from such case notes, here presented as clear and organised narratives. We must pay attention to how such material was disseminated and discussed, and how the categories present in published literature made their way back to the asylum recording books. We need also to look at the relationship between the science of medicine and the science of statistics, as well as that between statistics, legal reforms, and subsequent changes to practice, and, finally, we must also consider to what extent different practices transformed the nature of the knowledge that emerged from the asylum casebook and was translated into textbooks and journals. Late Victorian melancholia was constituted as a disorder of emotion chiefly characterised by 'depression', 'mental pain', 'suicidal propensities', and 'religious delusions'. In the last quarter of the nineteenth century the diagnosis was remarkably coherent and precise; however a comparison between published literature and asylum records illustrates the conflicts that arise and, consequently, the negotiations that must take place when medicine seeks to label and classify the complexities of human life.

NOTES

1. Thomas S. Clouston, *Clinical Lectures on Mental Diseases* (London: J. & A. Churchill, 1883), 35.
2. Royal Edinburgh Asylum, Male Casebooks, 1874–1875, Lothian Health Services Archives, Edinburgh University Library, Ref: LHB 7/51/25.
3. Joseph J. Brown, "Case of Determined Suicidal Melancholia," *Edinburgh Medical Journal* 20 (1874): 402.
4. Thomas S. Clouston, "Report of the Physician-Superintendent for the Year 1874," *Annual Report of the Royal Edinburgh Asylum for the Insane, Morningside, Royal Edinburgh Asylum* (1875), 15.
5. *Union Chargeability: A Bill to Provide for Better Distribution of Charge for Relief of Poor in Unions, House of Commons*, 1865, Vol. IV.607.
6. Clouston, "Report: 1874," 13.
7. In England and Wales, two physicians were required for private patients, one for paupers.
8. See e.g. Andrew Scull, ed., *Madhouses, Mad-Doctors, and Madmen: The Social History of Psychiatry in the Victorian Era* (Philadelphia: University of Pennsylvania Press, 1981), and *The Most Solitary of Afflictions: Madness and Society in Britain 1700–1900* (New Haven: Yale University Press, 1993); Anne Digby, *Madness, Morality, and Medicine: A Study of the York Retreat, 1796–1914* (Cambridge: Cambridge University Press, 1985); Bill Forsythe and Joseph Melling, *The Politics of Madness: The State, Insanity, and Society in England, 1845–1914* (London: Routledge, 2006); Charlotte McKenzie, *Psychiatry for the Rich: A History of Ticehurst Private Asylum, 1792–1917* (London: Routledge, 1992); David Wright, *Mental Disability in Victorian England: The Earlswood Asylum 1847–1901* (Oxford: Clarendon Press, 2001); Nancy Tomes, *A Generous Confidence: Thomas Story Kirkbride and the Art of Asylum Keeping, 1840–1883* (Cambridge: Cambridge University Press, 1984).
9. Scull, "The Social History of Psychiatry in the Victorian Era," in *Madhouses, Mad-Doctors, and Madmen*, 12–13.

10. Andrew Scull, *The Insanity of Place, the Place of Insanity: Essays on the History of Psychiatry* (London: Routledge, 2006), 110.
11. Ann Goldberg, *Sex, Religion and the Making of Modern Madness: The Eberbach Asylum and German Society, 1815–1849* (Oxford: Oxford University Press, 1999), 5.
12. Forsythe and Melling, *The Politics of Madness*.
13. Akihito Suzuki, "Framing Psychiatric Subjectivity: Doctor, Patient and Record-Keeping at Bethlem in the Nineteenth Century," in *Insanity, Institutions and Society, 1800–1914: A Social History of Madness in Comparative Perspective*, eds. Joseph Melling and Bill Forsythe (London: Routledge, 1999).
14. Anne Shepherd and David Wright, "Madness, Suicide, and the Victorian Asylum: Attempted Self-Murder in the Age of Non-Restraint," *Medical History* 46 (2002): 175–196.
15. Goldberg, *Making of Modern Madness*, 5.
16. Jonathan Andrews, Asa Briggs, Roy Porter, Penny Tucker, and Keir Waddington, *The History of Bethlem* (London and New York: Routledge, 1997); Alan Beveridge, "Madness in Victorian Edinburgh: A Study of Patients Admitted to the Royal Edinburgh Asylum under Thomas Clouston, 1873–1908: Part I & II," *History of Psychiatry* 6 (1995): 21–54, 133–156; Sarah Chaney, "Suicide, Mental Illness and the Asylum: The Case of Bethlem Royal Hospital, 1845–1875' (MA diss., University College London, 2009); McKenzie, *Psychiatry for the Rich*; Trevor Turner, *A Diagnostic Analysis of the Casebooks of Ticehurst House Asylum, 1845–1890* (Cambridge: Cambridge University Press, 1992).
17. Scottish Lunacy Commission, *Report by Her Majesty's Commissioners Appointed to Inquire into the State of Lunatic Asylums in Scotland*, Edinburgh, printed for Her Majesty's stationary office by Thomas Constable, 1857.
18. *Lunacy Act (Scotland)*, 1857. Its first chief medical commissioner was the reputable Scottish alienist W.A.F. Browne, father of James Crichton-Browne.
19. Thomas S. Clouston, "Report of the Physician-Superintendent for the Year 1876," *Annual Report of the Royal Edinburgh Asylum for the Insane, Morningside, Royal Edinburgh Asylum* (1877), 10–11.
20. David Kennedy Henderson, *The Evolution of Psychiatry in Scotland* (Edinburgh: E. & S. Livingstone, 1964), 93–93; Jonathan Andrews and Iain Smith, "The Evolution of Psychiatry in Glasgow during the Nineteenth and Early Twentieth Centuries," in *150 Years of British Psychiatry: Vol. 2: The Aftermath*, eds. German E. Berrios and Hugh Freeman (London: Athlone Press, 1996), 313; Alan Beveridge, "Madness in Victorian Edinburgh: A Study of Patients Admitted to the Royal

204   Å. JANSSON

Edinburgh Asylum under Thomas Clouston, 1873–1908: Part I," *History of Psychiatry* 6 (1995): 23–24.

21. (Author unknown) "Sir Thomas Smith Clouston: Obituary," *BMJ* (April 24, 1915): 744–746. That Clouston's obituary spanned almost three full pages in the *BMJ* (and was accompanied by a shorter piece by his protégé and successor, George Robertson) testifies to the prominent position he had achieved in the British medical community by the time of his death. Despite this, little has been written about the man himself by historians; however, a brief account can be found in Allan Beveridge, "Thomas Clouston and the Edinburgh School of Psychiatry," in *150 Years of British Psychiatry, 1841–1991*, eds. German E. Berrios and Hugh Freeman (London: Gaskell, 1991).

22. 'Thomas Laycock: Obituary," 448.

23. Thomas S. Clouston, "The Study of Mental Disease, being the Introductory Lecture Delivered in the University of Edinburgh, on the Institution of the Lectureship on Mental Diseases, May 1879," *Edinburgh Medical Journal* 25 (1879): 3.

24. George M. Robertson, *'The Hospitalisation of the Scottish Asylum System', The Presidential Address Delivered at the Annual Meeting Held in the Hall of the Royal College of Physicians, Edinburgh, on Wednesday, July 19, 1922* (London: Adlard & Son and West Newman, 1922).

25. David Skae, "A Rational and Practical Classification of Insanity," *Journal of Mental Science* 47 (1863): 311.

26. For a different kind of analysis of Clouston's reports than the one undertaken here, see Beveridge, "Madness in Victorian Edinburgh, Part I & II," 21–54, 133–156.

27. Thomas S. Clouston, "Report of the Physician-Superintendent for the Year 1873," *Annual Report of the Royal Edinburgh Asylum for the Insane, Morningside, Royal Edinburgh Asylum* (1874), n14–15.

28. Clouston, "Report: 1874," 15.

29. Beveridge, "Madness in Victorian Edinburgh, Part II," 135.

30. Clouston, "Report: 1874," 40.

31. Clouston, *Clinical Lectures*, 33–34. Emphasis in original. See also Thomas S. Clouston, "The Relationship of Bodily and Mental Pain," *Weekly Medical Review* 14 (1886): 600–609.

32. Clouston, *Clinical Lectures*, 35.

33. Clouston, *Clinical Lectures*, 37.

34. Clouston, *Clinical Lectures*, 38.

35. Clouston, *Clinical Lectures*, 38–40.

36. Clouston, *Clinical Lectures*, 40–41.

37. Clouston, *Clinical Lectures*, 64–79. Clouston did, however, also note the occasional 'untypical' case in his published material. See Thomas S. Clouston, "A Peculiar Case of Melancholia, with Cancerous Tumour

of the Middle Lobe of Brain, Disease of Kidneys, Liver, Pylorus, &c.,"
Journal of Mental Science 23, No. 104 (1878): 565–571.

38. Clouston, *Clinical Lectures*, 90–91.

39. Thomas S. Clouston, "On Mental Nursing," reprinted from *The Morn-ingside Mirror*, from three lectures delivered to asylum staff on 24 Nov 1887, Royal Edinburgh Asylum Staff Publications, Lothian Health Services Archives, University of Edinburgh, 2. *The Morningside Mirror* was the asylum's own publication, born after a printing press was installed at Morningside in 1845.

40. Clouston, *Clinical Lectures*, 107.

41. See Chapter 5.

42. Clouston, *Clinical Lectures*, 112.

43. John Harley Warner, "The Uses of Patient Records by Historians: Patterns, Possibilities, and Perplexities," *Health and History* 1, No. 2/3 (1999): 109.

44. Medical Certificates and Reception Order for Isabella Kay, admitted 31 July 1893, Lothian Health Services Archives, University of Edinburgh, Ref: LHB7/52/724.

45. Royal Edinburgh Asylum, Female Casebooks, June 1893–June 1894, Lothian Health Services Archives, University of Edinburgh, Ref: LHB7/51/60.

46. Royal Edinburgh Asylum, Female Casebooks, August 1876–April 1878, Lothian Health Services Archives, University of Edinburgh, Ref: LHB7/51/31.

47. Royal Edinburgh Asylum, Male Casebooks, October 1876–April 1878, Lothian Health Services Archives, University of Edinburgh, Ref: LHB7/51/30.

48. Royal Edinburgh Asylum, Female Casebooks, June 1893–June 1894, Lothian Health Services Archives, University of Edinburgh, Ref: LHB7/51/60.

49. Royal Edinburgh Asylum, Male Casebooks, July 1893–August 1894, Lothian Health Services Archives, University of Edinburgh, Ref: LHB7/51/61.

50. Female Casebook (Edinburgh), June 1893–June 1894.

51. Male Casebook (Edinburgh), July 1893–August 1894.

52. Royal Edinburgh Asylum, Female Casebooks, December 1897–December 1898, Lothian Health Services Archives, University of Edinburgh, Ref: LHB7/51/72.

53. David Walker and Anita O'Connell, "Introduction," in *Depression and Melancholy, 1660–1800, Vol 1: General Introduction & Religious Writings*, eds. Leigh Wetherall Dickson, Allan Ingram, David Walker, and Anita O'Connell (London: Pickering & Chatto, 2012).

54. Male Casebook (Edinburgh), October 1876–April 1878.

55. Female Casebook (Edinburgh), August 1876–April 1878.
56. Royal Edinburgh Asylum, Female Casebooks, April 1887–July 1888, Lothian Health Services Archives, University of Edinburgh, Ref: LHB7/51/48.
57. Royal Edinburgh Asylum, Male Casebooks, November 1887–March 1889, Lothian Health Services Archives, University of Edinburgh, Ref: LHB7/51/49.
58. Male Casebook (Edinburgh), October 1876–April 1878.
59. Female Casebook (Edinburgh), August 1876–April 1878.
60. Brookwood Female Casebook 1878–1880 Ref: 3043/5/9/2/11.
61. Female Casebook (Brookwood) 1878–1880.
62. Brookwood Male Casebook 1869–1872 Ref: 3043/5/9/1/2.
63. Thomas S. Clouston, "Physician-Superintendent's Annual Report for the Year 1887," *Annual Report of the Royal Edinburgh Asylum for the Insane, Morningside, Royal Edinburgh Asylum* (1888), 14.
64. Clouston, "Report: 1887," 41.
65. Female Casebook (Edinburgh), April 1887–July 1888.
66. Brown, "Suicidal Melancholia"; Royal Edinburgh Asylum, Male Casebooks, January 1874–April 1875, Lothian Health Services Archives, University of Edinburgh, Ref: LHB7/51/26.
67. Female Casebook (Edinburgh), August 1876–April 1878.
68. Female Casebook (Edinburgh), August 1876–April 1878; Male Casebook (Edinburgh), October 1876–April 1878; Female Casebook (Edinburgh), April 1887–July 1888.
69. Male Casebook (Edinburgh), November 1887–March 1889; Female Casebook (Edinburgh), June 1893–June 1894.
70. Male Casebook (Edinburgh), July 1893–August 1894.
71. Female Casebook (Edinburgh), December 1897–December 1898.
72. Female Casebook (Edinburgh), December 1897–December 1898; Female Casebook (Edinburgh), April 1887–July 1888; Male Casebook (Edinburgh), November 1887–March 1889.
73. Henry Maudsley, *The Pathology of Mind*, 3rd ed. (London: Macmillan, 1879), 384.
74. Brookwood Male Casebook 1869–1872 Ref: 3043/5/9/1/2.
75. Brookwood Female Casebooks 1868–1871 Ref: 3043/5/9/2/3.
76. Brookwood Male Casebook 1869–1872 Ref: 3043/5/9/1/2.
77. Pauper relief in Scotland was subject to the *Poor Law (Scotland) Act of 1845*, which had created a system similar to the English one implemented in 1834. For a more comprehensive discussion of the relationship between the Scottish pauper and lunacy laws, see Margaret Sorbie Thompson, "The Mad, the Bad, and the Sad: Psychiatric Care in the Royal Edinburgh Asylum (Morningside), 1813–1894" (PhD diss., Boston University, 1984), 18–31.

78. Female Casebook (Edinburgh), April 1887–July 1888.
79. Male Casebook (Edinburgh), November 1887–March 1889.
80. Clouston, *Clinical Lectures*, 107.
81. Thomas S. Clouston, "Report of the Physician-Superintendent for the Year 1879," *Annual Report of the Royal Edinburgh Asylum for the Insane, Morningside, Royal Edinburgh Asylum* (1880), 18–19.
82. Clouston, *Clinical Lectures*, 118.
83. Sarah Chaney, "Self-Control, Selfishness, and Mutilation: How Medical Is Self-Injury Anyway?" *Medical History* 55, No. 3 (2011): 377–380. See also Sarah Chaney, *Psyche on the Skin: A History of Self-Harm* (London: Reaktion Books), 2017.
84. See e.g. *Diagnostic and Statistical Manual for Mental Disorders, Fifth Edition (DSM-5)* (Washington, DC: The American Psychiatric Association, 2013), 803–805.
85. See Chaney, "Self-Control, Selfishness, and Mutilation," and *Psyche on the Skin*. For mid-twentieth-century psychiatric conceptions of 'attempted suicide', see Chris Millard, *A History of Self-Harm in Britain: A Genealogy of Cutting and Overdosing* (London: Palgrave Macmillan), 2015.

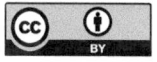

CHAPTER 7

Conclusion: Melancholia, Depression, and the Politics of Classification

Opinion is not the same thing as evidence, of course. Yet how to read the evidence on affective illness has proven highly contentious, while the momentum of opinion is clear for all to see.[1]

Edward Shorter (2007)

The only things that one really knows about human nature is that it changes.[2]

Oscar Wilde (1891)

This book has sought to map the reconceptualisation of melancholia as a modern biomedical mood disorder in nineteenth-century psychological medicine. In the first half of the century, physicians began to draw on experimental physiology to explain mental phenomena, creating a language and conceptual framework with which to describe emotional functionality. Central to this framework was the concept of psychological reflex action, which allowed physicians to explain emotion as an involuntary act that was both physiological and psychological. Within this context, melancholia was reconstituted as a disorder of emotion, a pathological state that arose when the brain was subjected to repeated irritation, over time affecting the tone of the cerebral tissue, resulting in pathological reflexive action. At this time, the nosological status of melancholia in British literature was uncertain, as several medical writers sought to replace it with, or subsume it under, other categories such as monomania. Towards the end of the century, however, melancholia was one of the

© The Author(s) 2021
Å Jansson, *From Melancholia to Depression*,
Mental Health in Historical Perspective,
https://doi.org/10.1007/978-3-030-54802-5_7

most frequently diagnosed conditions in British asylums, and the disorder was awarded considerable attention in diagnostic literature. Moreover, the internal biological model used to explain the disease, and the group of symptoms used to define and diagnose it, displayed remarkable coherence for its time.

The standardisation of melancholia in the second half of the nineteenth century occurred in a number of ways. First of all, the adoption by medical psychologists of a psycho-physiological framework for explaining mental disease facilitated a coherent internal model for this modern disease concept. Secondly, the argument that mental disease did not necessitate intellectual derangement but could be purely or largely affective became almost universally accepted within mid-century British medicine. Thirdly, following the creation of centralised bodies to oversee the implementation of lunacy law and the management of asylums, and the rapid growth of lunacy administration that followed, diagnostic and recording practices were increasingly standardised. Despite continued disagreement over nosology among Britain's asylum physicians, a de facto standardised system of classification emerged in which melancholia held a prominent position as an independent disease category. Finally, as a corollary of centralised lunacy administration and management, a large body of statistics was created containing every conceivable piece of information about Britain's asylum population. Statistical tables from around the country repeatedly suggested that melancholics were overwhelmingly suicidal, contributing to a homogenous symptom picture for melancholia in which suicidality was a defining criterion.

The story of how nineteenth-century biomedical melancholia was created and reified illustrates some of the inherent tensions within the psychiatric discipline, tensions that persist in the twenty-first century: on the one hand the conflict between biological disease models and descriptive nosologies, and on the other the uneasy relationship between neat medical categories and eclectic human life. The story of melancholia in this period constitutes only one small corner of psychiatric history, but it offers a window into the ways in which such medical knowledge about people is created and operates. As we saw in the final chapter, the people who were diagnosed with melancholia did not always fit so easily and neatly into this medical category. Rather, a multitude of different acts and expressions were merged into single keywords such as 'depression', 'mental pain', 'suicidal tendencies', and 'religious delusions'. Victorian physicians themselves acknowledged the difficulty in labelling and categorising with accuracy the vast array of human emotionality with which they met on asylum wards and in hospitals and private practices. Nevertheless, they repeatedly emphasised the necessity of psychiatric classification, no matter how flawed any such system was. In this way, they set the trend for psychiatric epistemology ever since.

ALTERNATIVE MODELS OF MELANCHOLIA

In 1901 psychiatrist Bernard Hollander published a lengthy article in the *Journal of Mental Science* titled 'The Cerebral Localisation of Melancholia' in which he argued that recent neurophysiological data suggested a specific location in the brain for this emotional disorder.[3] Hollander's theory of mind was in part based on a revised version of Franz Joseph Gall's early nineteenth-century phrenological system, which enjoyed a period of popularity among the reading public, but which had been widely discredited by scientists. A decade earlier Hollander had presented a paper to the Royal Anthropological Institute in which he argued that recent neurophysiological experiments, especially those conducted by David Ferrier, provided ample support for a revised, 'scientific', version of Gall's phrenology. Drawing upon Charles Darwin's *The Expression of the Emotions in Man and Animals* (1872),[4] Hollander suggested a strong link between facial expressions and emotional states. Following from this, he held that galvanic experiments on animals eliciting various muscular contractions in the face normally seen to correspond to specific emotions indicated that different feeling states could be induced by exciting different parts of the brain.[5]

This view was, Hollander argued, clearly supported by Ferrier's experiments in which electric currents had been applied to 'the ascending frontal convolution' in monkeys, dogs, and cats 'with the effect of elevating the cheeks and angles of the mouth with closure of the eyes'.[6] Hollander proceeded to quote a substantial section from Darwin's *Expression*, suggesting that when men and animals alike are experiencing 'high spirits' the corners of the mouth will inevitably and universally be drawn upwards. This observation in conjunction with Ferrier's physiological experiments led him to conclude that 'pleasurable emotions produce a nerve current, which takes its start in this region'.[7] Ferrier attended the session and partook in the discussion that followed from Hollander's presentation. According to the notes from the debate, Ferrier was generally in favour of the idea of localisation of various mental functions, but cautioned against conjectural leaps, suggesting that while Hollander's thesis begged consideration, present scientific research could not support his claims. However, Ferrier and the other attendants were in agreement that there may certainly be a future for more detailed and exact brain localisation of mental functions. The problem was how to proceed from the present vantage point to sound scientific explanation. Ferrier, in particular, suggested that while 'scientific phrenology might one day become possible', the route by which one could arrive at such a system must be staked out with care and precision.[8] Hollander's views on the localisation of melancholia were not widely appropriated at the time, but the attempts to locate emotion in specific parts of the brain have continued into the present.

Towards the end of World War I, Sigmund Freud published an article on 'mourning and melancholia' that offered a striking contrast to the biomedical model of the late nineteenth century, and to Hollander's neo-phrenological argument for the localisation of melancholia. Freud compared melancholia to mourning, noting that the two states of mind broadly shared the same features, but only the former was generally regarded as a form of illness. Mourning was for Freud a response to 'object-loss' and he conceptualised melancholia along the same lines, with one significant difference—in mourning, the loss of object was clear and the sufferer aware of it, but in melancholia the loss was unconsciously experienced. In other words, '[i]n mourning it is the world which has become poor and empty; in melancholia it is the ego itself'.[9] In this way, Freud brought attention to what had been perceived by Victorian physicians as their patients' (incorrect) assessment of their suffering—i.e. that it was without cause. The argument that pathological low mood could be distinguished from ordinary sadness or grief in part due to the absence of external cause was equally part of early-to-mid-twentieth-century descriptions of clinical depression. It must be noted, however, that this criterion was always an ambiguous one, an emotional trauma such as bereavement were often perceived to trigger disorder. On the question of causation, then, the boundary between ordinary and pathological sadness was never clear. And as will be seen momentarily, it was further obscured with the reconstitution of depressive illness as Major Depressive Disorder in the last quarter of the twentieth century.

FROM MELANCHOLIA TO DEPRESSION

Where, then, does the history of melancholia end and the history of depression begin? In the first decades of the twentieth century the use of melancholia as a diagnostic category rapidly declined. However, whether one writes the history of melancholia as a word, or as a concept or concepts, no clear-cut end point exists—as we saw in the Introduction, melancholia is inextricably linked to depression in contemporary literature, both psychiatric and historical. Moreover, the term melancholia has continued to feature peripherally in medical language throughout the twentieth and early twenty-first centuries, and both melancholy and melancholia appear with some regularity in the language and imagery of popular culture, literature, and philosophy.[10] However, the biomedical model of melancholia that reached its apex in British psychological medicine in the last three decades of the nineteenth century did not retain this prominent position for long, nor did it remain aetiologically and symptomatologically stable. With the emergence of an increasing number of conceptual frameworks for explaining the mind, and a growing separation of asylum and outpatient psychiatry, focus began to shift. Maudsley's argument in favour of bringing medical attention to bear upon what might be perceived as non-pathological emotional states came to inform practice and theory within the psy disciplines to an ever greater extent, particularly in the realm of psychoanalysis.

Two events at the turn of the twentieth century had significant repercussions for the classification and diagnosis of low mood. The first of these was the nosology introduced by Emil Kraepelin in 1899, in which he divided mental disorders into dementia praecox and manic-depressive insanity, that is, into a broadly cognitive illness and a broadly affective one. European psychiatrists had been gradually moving towards this kind of classification for some time. As we saw in Chapter 4, Maudsley had divided insanity into affective and ideational in 1867. In the early 1890s, Krafft-Ebing suggested that most forms of mental disorder could be separated into 'psychoneuroses' and 'psychic degenerations'. The former category included melancholia and mania, which he perceived as largely curable and with later onset, while the latter, which included constitutional affective insanity and paranoia, often appeared earlier in life and were more likely to become chronic. Kraepelin's subsequent division was, then, in part a rearticulation of existing knowledge. However, dementia praecox and manic-depressive insanity were classified as individual conditions with subtypes rather than as umbrella categories. This had important consequences for melancholia, which was largely done away with as a stand-alone category. Its symptoms were subsumed under manic-depressive insanity as a depressive stage, with the exception of 'involutional melancholia', a particular type of mood disorder that Kraepelin saw as affecting the elderly.[11]

Kraepelin's nosology proved hugely influential, both in the immediate years following its initial publication, as well as for the reform of psychiatric classification that occurred in the last quarter of the twentieth century with the arrival of *DSM-III*, the third edition of the APA's diagnostic manual. *DSM-III*, first published in 1980, has been referred to as 'neo-Kraepelinian'.[12] It endorsed a clear separation between affective and cognitive disorders, and presented a version of depressive illness in which many symptoms of melancholia, in particular delusions and hallucinations, were marginalised. 'Depression' had eclipsed (rather than replaced) melancholia as the major non-cyclical mood disorder by this point, a development that was set into motion in the first decade of the twentieth century. Kraepelin's dichotomy had threatened to all but erase melancholia from diagnostic literature, but the concept of a unitary depressive disorder was retained with the shift to a new term for this type of illness: depression.

At a 1905 meeting of the New York Neurological Society, Adolf Meyer had suggested that melancholia was not particularly useful as a diagnostic category, since the name 'implied a knowledge of something' that medicine 'did not possess'. He proposed to do away with it entirely, to be replaced by a symptomatic term that described one of the most tangible features of this illness:

> If, instead of melancholia, we applied the term depression to the whole class, it would designate in an unassuming way exactly what was meant by the common use of the term melancholia; and nobody would doubt that for medical purposes the term would have to be amplified so as to denote the kind of depression. In the large group of depressions we would naturally distinguish our cases according to aetiology, the symptom-complex, the course of the disease and the results.....The distinction had best be made according to the intrinsic nature of the depression. From that point of view we might distinguish the pronounced types from the simple insufficiently differentiated depressions.[13]

One must be careful not to suggest that melancholia became depression. There was no simple transition from one to the other, and the field of emotional disorders was further confounded by a focus on the 'war neuroses' of WWI.[14] There are many overlaps between the two categories, but they are not, and have never been, interchangeable. Kraepelin's and Meyer's classifications of low mood were influential and durable, and many early twentieth-century diagnostic texts incorporated elements of both. In this way, depression became cemented as an independent category alongside manic-depressive insanity. When the first edition of the *DSM* was published in 1952, a fusion of the two systems produced a nosology that echoed Maudsley's 1867 division of melancholia, whereby depression was divided into two types, a neurotic and a psychotic version. A similar division of depression had been presented in the WHO's *International Classification of Diseases (ICD)* in 1949. In the early post-war period, then, it was widely accepted within Anglo-American psychiatry that two types of depressions existed: a simple or neurotic form, and a melancholic or psychotic. *DSM-III* did away with this division with the introduction of 'Major Depressive Episode' (later also 'Disorder'). Today this ubiquitous mood disorder reigns supreme, but melancholia or melancholic depression has continued to exist alongside, and in an increasingly uneasy relationship with, the now more mainstream depressive illness favoured by the major diagnostic manuals. Standard depression is defined as low mood, loss of interest or pleasure, fatigue, bodily retardation, guilt or feelings of worthlessness, insomnia or hypersomnia, changes to appetite and body weight, and suicidality (symptoms must be present for at least two weeks). The most marked difference between depression so defined and melancholia is the absence of psychotic symptoms in the former. Since the arrival of *DSM-III*, these are retained only for a minor subtype, depression 'with melancholic features'.

This way of classifying low mood, which was maintained in the fifth (2013) edition of the *DSM*, has been subject to much critique both from within and outside the field of psychiatry.[15] One major criticism is that the category Major Depressive Disorder is too broad, and that its criteria blurs the boundary between normal and pathological low mood. The *DSM-III* task force did away with a previous 'bereavement exclusion' qualifier, meaning that depression was no longer distinguished from ordinary low mood by the absence of cause. Moreover, the period for which symptoms had to manifest for a diagnosis was shortened from one month to two weeks. These decisions led critics to argue that the category depression has been expanded to the point of becoming largely useless.[16]

The second criticism of Major Depressive Disorder concerns the decision of the APA to endorse a single unitary depression instead of the two types referred to above. Edward Shorter argues that this was not a decision based on scientific evidence. Rather, he suggests, the *DSM-III* task force had originally intended to include a 'minor' and 'major' depression in the new manual, but felt under pressure to drop the former as 'insurance companies would never pay for anything "minor"'.[17] As discussed in the Introduction, advocates of the two depressions model continue to argue for the reinstatement in diagnostic literature of a second, more severe form of psychotic or melancholic depression, which is defined both in terms of mental and physical symptoms and specific biological markers. Shorter and colleagues argue that the key to such a definition of melancholia—one that is both clinically and biologically reliable—lies with a combination of symptomatological descriptions (a statistically based system) and measurable biological markers (a physiological foundation). Shorter has contributed a historical perspective as one of the key building blocks of the case for the resurrection of melancholia. His narrative is one in which 'biological psychiatry' was founded in the nineteenth century and has continued to develop along a progressive (albeit bumpy) path ever since.[18] In 2007, the year after the Copenhagen conference discussed in the Introduction, Shorter published a book together with Conrad Swartz on 'psychotic depression', which presented a more detailed version of the argument for an endocrine-based definition of melancholia. The marginalisation of endocrinal research in psychiatry, they argue, has occurred to the detriment of this branch of medical science, as it holds the key to a greater understanding of mental disorders.[19] Shorter and colleagues are far from alone in the desire to—finally—make psychiatry truly biological. When work on the fifth edition of the *DSM* was still ongoing, the head of the US National Institute for Mental Health argued that such a reconstitution of psychiatric classification is essential because '[p]atients with mental disorders deserve better'.[20] This line of argument is significant; a system of classification that recognises the biological (neurological, genetic, endocrinal) basis of mental disorders is in the best interest of the people who are perceived to be suffering from such conditions.

However, advocates for the 'resurrection' of melancholia as a distinct mood disorder with biological markers also point to historical evidence in making their argument, suggesting that melancholia is a universal, timeless condition that has always existed. The temptation to draw on history to legitimise current psychiatric knowledge is obvious, but it is both unhelpful and unnecessary. The question is not so much whether or not we *can* plausibly diagnose people in the past with current conditions and vice versa, but rather, whether we should. What is gained by doing so? Does it serve its intended purpose, that is, if we can show that people have suffered from the same illness throughout history, does this affirm that the condition is real? It is difficult to see how it does. Historical records tell us nothing about the experience, psychopathology, or biological reality of people in the present. The current empirical data that forms the basis of arguments for a distinct melancholic depression is convincing, and if the APA and the WHO agreed to formally recognise melancholia as presently described, this could potentially benefit people suffering from severe low mood with psychotic and pronounced bodily symptoms, in terms of swifter access to more appropriate treatment. One might argue, then, that there is an urgent need to formally accept the validity of a melancholic depression as a distinct diagnosis. But it does not follow that this is done by demonstrating universality across time. The idea that this is a possible and plausible approach to scientific knowledge echoes a Baconian perception of 'nature' as something that human beings can observe, intervene with, and learn from, and about which universal truths can be demonstrated. But this idea of nature is itself historically specific. And moreover, the scientific method cannot be applied to long-dead historical subjects whom we believe to have suffered from melancholia, nor to the documents they have left behind.

Current medico-scientific knowledge about melancholia does not gain its validity and legitimacy from its presumed timelessness and universality. Rather, if it is a valid and legitimate diagnosis reflecting the experience of living subjects in the present, it is precisely because it is real right now. Projecting it onto past and long gone individuals who are only names on papers does not help to make it more 'true' in the present. What it does, however, is threaten to demote history from its place as a rich, constructive, and critical human science, a science that offers a different kind of insight, by showing how things change, and how knowledge is produced, instead reducing it to a one-dimensional discipline, the main task of which is to lend legitimacy to current knowledge within the natural sciences. When it comes to medical knowledge about the emotional life of humans, we might do better to distinguish the past from the present. Much can learnt about each from the other, but there is little to be gained from attempting to equate the two. This does not diminish current knowledge about melancholic depression. What we know today is not any less valuable or helpful because it applies only to the present and not the past. When it comes to treating people, to alleviating severe and debilitating low mood, it is our actions in the present and the future that matter. This is the real value of medical knowledge—what we can do with it right now.

The real value of history is not as a legitimising tool for such knowledge, rather it is to show how present knowledge (medical or any other) was created, and in this way help us gain a broader, deeper, and richer understanding of the human condition. This should not be taken as a rejection of biological claims about human beings. The aim here is not to replace scientific conceptions of self, of mind and emotions, with historical ones. The division between the human and the natural sciences is equally historically constituted[21]; these different 'sciences' represent different ways of knowing ourselves and our world, a multitude of 'partial perspectives'.[22] Rather than foregrounding one as the source of truth, a more hopeful approach would be to consider the wealth of knowledge at our disposal when we are able to allow for multiple epistemologies. The antagonistic relationship often perceived between the natural sciences and the humanities is both unnecessary and unhelpful. What we might better strive for is an 'affirmative relationship' between these spheres, a relationship that, in the words of Nikolas Rose

> seeks to identify and work with those arguments that recognize, in whatever small way, the need for a new and non-reductionist biology of human beings and other organisms in their milieu, and which can thus be brought into conversation with the evidence, concepts and forms of analysis developed in the social and human sciences.[23]

THE POLITICS OF PATHOLOGICAL EMOTIONALITY

There are further reasons for promoting a more flexible, multidisciplinary, and multifaceted view of what it means to be human and of our emotional life. Medical approaches to low mood have undergone a number of significant shifts over the last two hundred years, one of which has been the focus of this book. Another was the rise of social models of depression in the mid-twentieth century,[24] which emerged in the context of the construction of the post-war Keynesian welfare state. In contrast to this, twenty-first-century biological approaches to emotion and its disorders can be seen as closely wedded to a neoliberal worldview. The link between socio-economic inequality and psychological distress such as depressed mood is widely acknowledged,[25] yet the dominant treatment for depression relies on the perception of pathological low mood as an individual problem of neurochemistry and emotional dysregulation. Clinical guidelines favour functional and cost-effective and/or profitable treatment approaches geared towards getting people back to work, specifically Cognitive Behavioural Therapy (CBT) and antidepressant medication.[26] Much has been written on the relationship between contemporary models of depression and the rise of antidepressants on the one hand, and neoliberal capitalism on the other.[27] The central aim of CBT and its sister therapy Dialectical Behaviour Therapy (DBT), emotion regulation, must equally be understood within the context of political economy.[28]

The pre-twentieth-century origins of emotion regulation have received scant attention by historians. As this book has shown, in the Victorian period a belief that most forms of insanity commenced with emotional disturbance was widely held among British physicians. Related to this was the view that many lunatics could not be held responsible for their actions.[29] The disordered emotions of the insane and the acts resulting from these (such as suicide) were not to be morally condemned, but biologically explicated and medically treated. Yet at the same time, physicians such as Henry Maudsley held that the development of pathological emotionality could be prevented through conscious individual effort. Persistent practice to monitor and master one's emotions would over time result in the formation of a healthy mind and moral conduct.[30] The idea that insanity could be prevented and that the development of a healthy mind was an individual duty was underpinned by a cultural framework where self-help and individual responsibility were celebrated virtues, and where 'freewill' was a powerful philosophical and political concept.[31]

This cultural framework has seen a resurgence in the age of neoliberalism.[32] The efficacy of the neoliberal programme is in part resulting from the ability of its proponents to successfully promote it as a non-ideological, rational, 'common sense' approach to economics and the organisation of society.[33] Over the last four decades, the core principles of neoliberalism have come to permeate every facet of human existence. Rose explains the subtle and effective ways in which what he refers to as 'advanced liberalism' has become an integral part of contemporary life, creating a society in which 'the regulation of public conduct' is closely linked to and underpinned by 'the subjective emotional and intellectual capacities and techniques of individuals, and the ethical regimes through which they govern their lives'.[34] Psychiatric and psychological strategies aimed at regulating pathological emotion and behaviour are one such ethical regime. In Britain today, the programme of individual self-help promoted by cognitive behavioural strategies is situated within a Conservative approach to welfare that measures an individual's health or illness in terms of their ability to perform productive work.[35] Both CBT and DBT are seen as functional and cost-effective strategies,[36] and a key goal of these at present is to return the individual to active society—and to paid labour—by treating the symptoms of mental distress in isolation from their wider social causes. Meanwhile, illustrating the paradoxes of the present system, government policies aimed at incentivising people to return to work have been shown to be a major cause of psychological distress, at times so profound it causes individuals to take their own lives.[37]

How are we to make sense of and address depression and melancholia in this context? In the first instance, the presently dominant way of classifying low mood sits well within the current economic framework. Major Depressive Disorder, as currently defined, constitutes a collection of symptoms that are perceived to respond well to standard antidepressant medication and CBT. Melancholic depression, which is seen as requiring different and more comprehensive psychiatric care and treatment, fits less comfortably in this context. This brings us to the problem of 'correct' classification in psychiatry, which has been a central theme of this book. As the present story illustrates, there is nothing natural or inevitable about how psychiatry defines, labels, and classifies human emotionality. Many of the decisions made about the classification of melancholia in the nineteenth century were the result of administrative concerns and the need to make diagnostic practices more efficient in the context of expanding asylum populations and limited resources. Similarly, the decision by the *DSM-III* task force to do away with a more severe, melancholic depression was at least in part motivated by financial concerns. It is perhaps unavoidable that nosological decisions will be driven not only by a desire for correct diagnosis and suitable treatment, but also by various political factors. There is no conclusive evidence regarding the former, and the latter includes many powerful forces, such as insurance providers and pharmaceutical companies.

While persistent conflicts and disagreement over how to classify mental disorders have plagued the psychiatric profession since its infancy, there has nevertheless been overwhelming support for the argument that classification is necessary. Critique of the usefulness and benevolence of classification is, however, growing, both from within and outside the psy disciplines. It has been suggested that the 'poor validity' of psychiatric diagnostics and the expansion of diagnostic categories to include an increasingly wide range of human behaviour cause more harm than good to the people whom psychiatry is meant to help, and that the current system of classifying psychological distress as specific mental disorders would be better replaced with an 'operational definition of different experiences and phenomena' without denoting clusters of these as specific disorders.[38] Callard and Bracken have highlighted some of the ways in which psychiatric labelling can be harmful. These include 'diagnostic overshadowing', whereby an existing psychiatric diagnosis can lead to the patient's physical symptoms being automatically attributed to that diagnosis, precluding a full medical investigation of those symptoms, as well as the long-term institutionalisation that can result from some types of psychiatric diagnoses. They conclude that diagnosis in psychiatry on the whole does more harm than good, and that 'the [mental health] interventions that have arguably empowered people the most, such as innovative community services, have not been diagnosis specific'.[39] Cooke and Kinderman have furthermore drawn attention to the problem of stigmatisation. Their critique centres on the schizophrenia diagnosis and the stigma attached to this psychiatric label, which in their view renders an already vulnerable group of people even more so. Adding to this are the 'feelings of hopelessness' that can result from being diagnosed with what is largely seen as a 'chronic' mental illness.[40]

The latter concern speaks to the complex and sometimes harmful relationship between psychiatric diagnosis and identity. Arguments for parity between physical and mental health often turn to current biological models of psychiatric illness to suggest that these two areas of pathology should be treated the same because they are the same—in this way, depression is no different from cancer or a broken leg. However, parity does not have to be based in sameness. On the contrary, such arguments are potentially harmful. In the first instance, psychiatric illness concerns the part of us that is most central to our personhood—the mind. While we continue to debate social and biological causes of mental distress, the ways in which such distress manifests are primarily (but not only) psychological and consequently also relational and identity-based, in ways that a broken leg is not. Attempts to frame mental disorders in strictly biological terms carry the risk of imprinting human beings in all their complexity with simplistic, reductionist biological stamps, which can potentially have a self-perpetuating effect. Secondly, as people internalise their diagnoses, this can feed back into, and reinforce, psychiatric labels (what Ian Hacking called 'looping effects'[41]). And finally, following from this, attempts to destigmatise 'mental illness' by framing psychiatric conditions as chiefly biological and to be equated with other medical conditions can lead people to feel 'less optimistic about their ability to get better' and increase public 'perceptions of dangerousness and unpredictability' of such disorders.[42]

At the same time, we must be careful not to simply reject existing diagnoses as not 'real' or 'true'. If depression exists in psychiatric literature as a mental illness, if people are diagnosed with this condition, and if they consequently experience themselves as 'having depression' or 'being depressed', then depression is inevitably a real thing. Moreover, framing one's suffering in medico-scientific terms is undoubtedly helpful for many people, especially in terms of alleviating feelings of guilt, shame, and personal responsibility. A more helpful and nuanced approach then, as we think about the future of psychological distress and psychiatric diagnostics, is to accept and validate both the concept and experience of 'depression' or 'melancholia' and other diagnoses as legitimate medical conditions, while at the same time allowing equal space for other explanations for and ways of naming difficult psychological experiences. And finally, it is imperative that we continue to argue forcefully for a comprehensive and multifaceted model of psychological distress that places human suffering in the context of material reality. A strict framing of severe and debilitating low mood as an internal problem, with the pathology located solely in the individual, marginalises critical approaches to the social and economic causes of emotional distress, and excludes political solutions to a problem that is increasingly shown to at least in part be the product of ideological decisions.

CONCLUSION

This book has mapped the reconstitution of melancholia as a modern biomedical mental disease in Victorian psychological medicine. It has tried to show how this medical category was created and reified through a combination of ideas and practices, which were specific to their temporal and cultural context. At the same time, however, many of the concepts that emerged through the creation of biomedical melancholia continue to inform current perceptions of emotion as a biological event that is subject to pathologisation. There are undoubtedly many similarities between nineteenth-century melancholia and our time's depression, as well as between these two conditions and earlier forms of melancholy and melancholia. But similarities across time should not be mistaken for inevitability. One must be careful to avoid falling into teleological traps when approaching historical events. When stories of people in the past appear familiar to the twenty-first-century reader, such familiarity is at least partly read into past accounts by those who are doing the reading. History is made now, in the present. By arguing for universality of human experiences based on current knowledge frameworks, the possibility for different accounts not just of the past but also of the present and the future are potentially foreclosed. As this book has aimed to show, the idea of pathological emotionality, of 'mood disorders', is historically specific. It was once created, made—which consequently implies that it can be unmade. This is where history becomes more than storytelling or academic pursuit. It shows that things can change, including the possibilities and limits of human experience. History, then, holds the promise of hope, of a future different from both the present and the past.

NOTES

1. Edward Shorter, "The Doctrine of the Two Depressions in Historical Perspective," *Acta Psychiatrica Scandinavica*, 115, S43: 5.
2. Oscar Wilde, *The Soul of Man under Socialism* (The Floating Press, 2009 [1891]), 51.
3. Bernard Hollander, "The Cerebral Localisation of Melancholia," *Journal of Mental Science* 47 (1901): 458–485.
4. Charles Darwin, *The Expression of the Emotions in Man and Animals* (London: J. Murray, 1872).

5. Bernard Hollander, "A Demonstration of Centres of Ideation in the Brain from Observation and Experiment," *Journal of the Anthropological Institute of Great Britain and Ireland* 19 (1890): 13. Hollander's localisation theory was provided with further rationale in the form of changes observed in patients following surgery to treat brain injuries, which he suggested indicated the specific localisation of melancholia in the parietal lobe, confirming that it was chiefly an emotional rather than an intellectual disorder. Bernard Hollander, "Can Insanity Be Cured by Surgical Operation?" *The Phrenologist* 6 (1907): 53–59.
6. Hollander, "A Demonstration," 15. See also Tiffany Watt-Smith on how Darwin's concept of the 'flinch' as an 'emotional gesture' reflected wider Victorian perceptions of the external manifestations of feeling: "Darwin's Flinch: Sensation Theatre and Scientific Looking in 1872," *Journal of Victorian Culture* 15, No. 1 (2010): 101–117.
7. Hollander, "A Demonstration," 15.
8. Cited in Hollander, "A Demonstration," 24–25 ('Discussion').
9. Sigmund Freud, "Mourning and Melancholia," reprinted in *The Standard Edition of the Complete Works of Sigmund Freud, Volume XIV (1914–1916)*, eds. James Strachey and Anna Freud (London: The Hogarth Press, 1957), 243–246 (quotation p. 246).
10. For instance, Danish director Lars von Trier named his film about depression as a metaphorical Armageddon 'Melancholia'. See also e.g. Julia Kristeva, *Black Sun: Depression and Melancholia* (New York: Columbia University Press, 1989).
11. Emil Kraepelin, *Psychiatrie: Ein Lehrbuch für Studirende und Aertze*, II Band, 6 Aufl. (Leipzig: J.A. Barth, 1899), 317–318. In the (abbreviated) English version of the textbook, the subcategory is translated as 'involutional melancholia'. Emil Kraepelin, *Clinical Psychiatry: A Text-Book for Students and Physicians*, 6th ed. (New York: Macmillan, 1904), 254.
12. Tayla Greene, "The Kraepelinian Dichotomy: The Twin Pillars Crumbling?," *History of Psychiatry* 18, No. 3 (2007): 361–379.
13. Adolf Meyer, quoted in "Proceedings of the New York Neurological Society," *Journal of Nervous and Mental Disease* 32, No. 2 (1905): 114.
14. e.g. Rhodri Hayward, "Sadness in Camberwell: Imagining Stress and Constructing History in Post-War Britain," in *Stress, Trauma and Adaptation in the Twentieth Century*, eds. David Cantor and Edmund Ramsden (Rochester, NY: Rochester University Press, 2012); Christopher M. Callaghan and German E. Berrios, *Reinventing Depression: A History of the Treatment of Depression in Primary Care, 1940–2004* (Oxford: Oxford University Press, 2005).
15. E.g. Thomas Insel et al., "Research Domain Criteria (RDoC): Toward a New Classification Framework for Research on Mental Disorders," *American Journal of Psychiatry* 167, No. 7 (2010): 748–751; Andy

Coghlan and Sarah Reardon, "Psychiatry Divided as Mental Health 'Bible' Denounced," *New Scientist*, 3 May 2013, http://www.newsci entist.com/article/dn23487-psychiatry-divided-as-mental-health-bible-denounced.html#.UhSi4z-1tBE. See also Mark Moran, "Continuity and Changes Mark New Text of DSM-5," *Psychiatric News*, 18 January 2013, http://psychnews.psychiatryonline.org/newsarticle.aspx?articleid= 1558423.

16. Allan V. Horwitz and Jerome C. Wakefield, *The Loss of Sadness: How Psychiatry Transformed Normal Sorrow into Depressive Disorder* (Oxford: Oxford University Press, 2007), 95–103.

17. Edward Shorter, *How Everyone Became Depressed: The Rise and Fall of the Nervous Breakdown* (Oxford: Oxford University Press, 2013), 134–135.

18. Edward Shorter, *A History of Psychiatry: From the Era of the Asylum to the Age of Prozac* (New York: Wiley, 1997).

19. Conrad M. Swartz and Edward Shorter, *Psychotic Depression* (Cambridge: Cambridge University Press, 2007).

20. Thomas Insel, "Director's Blog: Transforming Diagnosis," National Institute for Mental Health, 29 April 2013, http://www.nimh.nih.gov/ about/director/2013/transforming-diagnosis.shtml.

21. Roger Smith, *Being Human: Historical Knowledge and the Creation of Human Nature* (Manchester: Manchester University Press, 2007), Chapter 3.

22. Donna Haraway, "Situated Knowledges: The Science Question in Feminism and the Privilege of Partial Perspective," *Feminist Theory* 14, No. 3 (1988): 575–599.

23. Nikolas Rose, "The Human Sciences in a Biological Age," *Theory, Culture & Society* 30, No. 3 (2013): 24. At a time when interdisciplinarity is all the rage, it is worth considering the practical, political, and ethical challenges of collaboration between the natural, human, and social sciences. Callard and Fitzgerald draw on their own experience of interdisciplinary collaboration to shed light on and interrogate the object that is interdisciplinarity, asking what is at work—and at stake—when researchers from different epistemological traditions come together. Felicity Callard and Des Fitzgerald, *Rethinking Interdisciplinarity across the Social Sciences and Neurosciences* (Basingstoke: Palgrave Macmillan, 2015).

24. Hayward, "Sadness in Camberwell".

25. A wealth of research across disciplines suggest a link between socioeconomic inequality and depression (as well as other mental health conditions). See for instance: Vincent Lorant, et al., "Socioeconomic Inequalities in Depression: A Meta-Analysis," *American Journal of Epidemiology* 157, No. 2 (2003): 98–112.

26. See e.g. "Depression in Adults: Recognition and Management," National Institute for Health and Care Excellence (October 2009, last updated

April 2018). For a critique of policy approaches to depression in the age of neoliberalism (using Canada as an example), see Katherine Teghtsoonian, "Depression and Mental Health in Neoliberal Times: A Critical Analysis of Policy and Discourse," *Social Science & Medicine* 69, No. 1 (2009): 28–35.

27. See e.g. Joanna Moncrieff, "Psychiatric Drug Promotion and the Politics of Neoliberalism," *British Journal of Psychiatry* 188 (2006): 301–302.

28. Åsa Jansson, "Teaching 'Small and Helpless' Women How to Live: Dialectical Behaviour Therapy in Sweden, ca 1995–2005," *History of the Human Sciences* 31, No. 4 (2018): 131–157. DBT was developed specifically to treat (primarily women) diagnosed with Borderline Personality Disorder who were perceived to engage in suicidal and self-harming behaviour. It places significant emphasis on self-help and individual responsibility, and has been framed as a cost-effective strategy to treat a group of patients among whom the prevalence of in-patient care was traditionally high. In this context, it is also important to note, as Chris Millard does, that 'neoliberalism's stress on individual actors' radical freedom to make choices for their own benefit fits well with a model of self-harm that emphasises the individualistic, private feelings of tension, and the self-regulation of these through cutting'. Chris Millard, *A History of Self-Harm in Britain: A Genealogy of Cutting and Overdosing* (London: Palgrave Macmillan, 2015), 205.

29. This view, which remained controversial and contested throughout the Victorian period, formed the basis of the insanity defence, institutionalised following the M'Naghten trial of 1843. The argument was, however, subject to much disagreement both within and outside of the medical community. For an excellent look at the discussions on insanity and legal responsibility, see Roger Smith, *Trial by Medicine: Insanity and Responsibility in Victorian Trials* (Edinburgh: Edinburgh University Press, 1981), esp. pp. 14–17 for the M'Naghten rules.

30. See e.g. Henry Maudsley, *Body and Will* (New York: D. Appleton & Co, 1870), 93.

31. Roger Smith, *Free Will and the Human Sciences in Britain, 1870–1910* (London: Pickering and Chatto, 2013).

32. By this I mean the period from the late 1970s/early 1980s onward, when Keynesian economics were gradually abandoned in the West in favour of a neoliberal approach, which also came to be reflected in the policy orientation of international institutions such as the IMF, and forced upon much of the Global South through Western economic dominance both within and outside of institutional frameworks.

33. Stuart Hall in part attributes this to British pragmatism: Stuart Hall, "The Neo-Liberal Revolution," *Cultural Studies* 25, No. 6 (2011): 705–728.

See also Nick Srnicek and Alexander Williams, *Inventing the Future: Post-capitalism and a World without Work* (London: Verso, 2016), 60–64, who refer to neoliberalism as 'the single most successful hegemonic project of the last fifty years'.

34. Nikolas Rose, "Government, Authority and Expertise in Advanced Liberalism," *Economy and Society* 22, No. 3 (1993): 286–287.

35. For a critical analysis of the Work Capability Assessments see Benjamin Barr et al., "'First, Do No Harm': Are Disability Assessments Associated with Adverse Trends in Mental Health? A Longitudinal Ecological Study," *Journal of Epidemiology and Community Health* 70 (2016): 339–345.

36. See e.g. Sandra Hollinghurst et al., "Cost-Effectiveness of Therapist-Delivered Online Cognitive-Behavioural Therapy for Depression: Randomised Controlled Trial," *The British Journal of Psychiatry* 197, No. 4 (2010): 297–304; Roy Krawitz and Erin M. Miga, "Financial Cost Effectiveness of Dialectical Behaviour Therapy (DBT) for Borderline Personality Disorder (BPD)," in *The Oxford Handbook of Dialectical Behaviour Therapy*, ed. Michaela A. Swales (Oxford: Oxford University Press, 2018); Franske J. van Apeldoorn et al., "Cost-Effectiveness of CBT, SSRI, and CBT + SSRI in the Treatment for Panic Disorder," *Acta Psychiatrica Scandinavica* 129, No. 4 (2013): 286–295.

37. "Mental Health Discrimination 'Built into' Work Capability Assessment," Heriot Watt University, 23 February 2017, https://www.hw.ac.uk/news/articles/2017/mental-health-discrimination-built-into-work.htm. For a comprehensive analysis and critique of the link between suicide and austerity driven policies underpinned by neoliberal ideology see China Mills, "'Dead People Don't Claim': A Psychopolitical Autopsy of UK Austerity Suicides," *Critical Social Policy* 38, No. 2: 302–322.

38. Peter Kinderman, John Read, Joanna Moncrieff, and Richard Bentall, "Drop the Language of Disorder," *Evidence-Based Mental Health* 16 (2013): 2–3.

39. Felicity Callard, Pat Bracken, Anthony Davies, and Norman Santorius, "Has Psychiatric Diagnosis Labelled Rather Than Enabled Patients?" *BMJ*, 347 (2013): 4312–4313.

40. Anne Cooke and Peter Kinderman, "'But What About Real Mental Illnesses?' Alternatives to the Disease Model Approach to 'Schizophrenia'," *Journal of Humanistic Psychology* 58, No. 1 (2017): 58–59.

41. Ian Hacking, "The Looping Effects of Human Kinds," in *Causal Cognition: A Multidisciplinary Debate*, eds. Dan Sperber, David Premack, and Ann James Premack (Oxford: Clarendon Press, 1995).

42. Ashok Malla, Ridha Joober, and Amparo Garcia, "'Mental Illness Is Like Any Other Medical Illness': A Critical Examination of the Statement and Its Impact on Patient Care and Society," *Journal of Psychiatry & Neuroscience* 40, No. 3 (2015): 147–150.

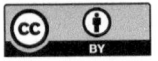

INDEX

© The Editor(s) (if applicable) and The Author(s) 2021
Å Jansson, *From Melancholia to Depression*,
Mental Health in Historical Perspective,
https://doi.org/10.1007/978-3-030-54802-5

Scottish Board of Commissioners, 140
Scott, Joan W., 32, 86, 170
self-mutilation, 200
Senhouse, William, 52, 60
Shorter, Edward, 209, 216, 223, 225
simple, 94, 95, 98, 109, 113, 114,
  117
simple melancholia, 151, 158, 159,
  162, 185
Skae, David, 175, 180, 181, 183,
  188, 204
Smith, Roger, 37, 38, 56, 164, 169
Solly, Samuel, 43, 44, 58
somnambulism, 51
Spencer, Herbert, 90, 92, 99, 100,
  115, 159, 169
statistics, 2, 7, 17, 32, 124, 127, 128,
  132, 133, 135–142, 144, 158,
  165–167, 210
suicidal/suicidality, 1, 11, 20, 23,
  108, 110, 112, 114, 124–128,
  133, 135, 139–143, 148,
  151, 154–160, 162, 163, 167,
  173–176, 182, 183, 185–187,
  189–200, 202, 210, 215

T
Taylor, Michael A., 4, 25, 26
temperament (melancholic), 65, 70,
  73, 75, 108
thermodynamics, 112
1845 Acts, 141, 166
Ticehurst private licensed house
  (Sussex), 176, 193, 202

tone (of the brain), 8, 10, 22, 39, 72,
  76, 92, 100, 103, 131, 147
Tuke, Daniel Hack, 67, 80, 81, 84,
  86–88, 104, 113, 119, 156

U
Union of Chargeability Act (1865),
  174
unitary psychosis, 94, 114, 116
the unpardonable sin, 127, 149, 150,
  153

V
van Deusen E.H., 111
Verwey, Gerlof, 92, 115, 116
volition, 40, 41, 47, 48, 52, 53, 55,
  59, 91, 95, 99, 101, 102, 106,
  116, 118

W
Wakefield Asylum (West Riding
  Pauper Asylum), 31, 158
war neuroses, 215
Wilcox, Arthur, 156
Williams, Joseph, 74, 75, 86
Winslow, Forbes, 139
workhouse, 135, 141, 142, 178, 193
World Health Organisation, 2
Wynn's Act, 133

Z
Zeller, Alfred, 91, 94, 116